The Biology of Beating Stress

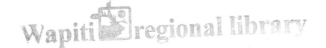
The Biology of Beating Stress

*How Changing Your Environment,
Your Body, and Your Brain Can Help
You Find Balance and Peace*

By
Jeanne Ricks, CHC

New Page Books
A Division of The Career Press, Inc
Pompton Plains, NJ

THE BIOLOGY OF BEATING STRESS
Cover design by Howard Grossman
Printed in the U.S.A.

To order this title, please call toll-free 1-800-CAREER-1 (NJ and Canada: 201-848-0310) to order using VISA or MasterCard, or for further information on books from Career Press.

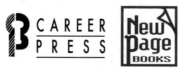

The Career Press, Inc.
220 West Parkway, Unit 12
Pompton Plains, NJ 07444
www.careerpress.com
www.newpagebooks.com

Library of Congress Cataloging-in-Publication Data
Ricks, Jeanne, 1961-
   The biology of beating stress : how changing your environment, your body, and your brain can help you find balance and peace/Jeanne Ricks.
      pages cm
   Includes bibliographical references and index.
   ISBN 978-1-60163-330-9 (pbk.) -- ISBN 978-1-60163-450-4 (ebook) 1. Stress management. 2. Respiration. 3. Exercise. 4. Self-care, Health. I. Title.
   RA785.R53 2014
   155.9'042--dc23

2014003196

For my parents, who taught me invaluable lessons
of strength and courage. They also shared with me a
tremendous appreciation for the music of language and
its power to communicate and create change.

Appreciations

I would like to thank my family of friends who constantly amaze me with their support and love.

Thank you to my advance readers: Lisa Fischer, Edna Williams, Delia McVoy, and Terri Rossi.

Many colleagues and friends directly and indirectly helped in the writing of this book: my Uncle Percy E. Ricks, Jill Clarke, Bill Weinberg, Jeanne Fletcher Mallette, Johnny "Ananda" Norman, Charles Walton, Kim Walton, Thomas C. Washington, Pamela Nunes, Evette Murray, Richard P. Stone, Paul Arnold, Frances Connor, Dorette Brown, Miguel Broom, Mark Brooks, Ehryck Gilmore, Paulette de Suzia, Robert Irving III, Eddie Maldonado, Chan, Veronica & Victoria Johnson, Studs Terkel, Joseph Campbell, Howard Thurman, Linus Pauling, Bruce Lipton, Candace Pert, Debbie Ford, Deepak Chopra, Joseph Mercola, Babette Rothschild, Larry Dossey, Brian L. Weiss, Panache Desai, Rupert Sheldrake, Gary Robert Buchanan, Roger K. Pitman, Ann Albers, Edwina Kee, Beth Dobrish, Jacqueline de Vries, Sheryl Levanthal, Sandy Beltramini, Sharon Mackey-McGee, Karen Mackey-Witherspoon, Keith Collins, Denise Richardson, Bob McCarthy; Neville Gupta, Mary Ann Donoghue, Christian Villalba, Ella Britton Gibson and many others too numerous to name here, but whom I hope know that I am grateful for their friendship and support.

Special thanks to Lisa Hagan of Paraview Literary Agency for her professionalism and attentive care. I thank also my publisher, Career Press Books, and their staff, who has shown such support and enthusiasm.

Last but not least, my thanks to you the readers around the world who make all of our efforts worthwhile.

Contents

7

Anxiety (or Dance With the Elephants) *100*

8

Meditation (Your Mini-Vacation) *124*

9

Brainwave Entrainment *128*

10

Sleep (Get More!) *136*

Author's Note

The information provided in this book, by necessity, is of a general nature and not a substitute for an evaluation or treatment by a competent medical specialist. It is sold with the understanding that the author and the publisher are not engaged in medical, psychological, legal, accounting, or other professional services. The dietary and supplemental suggestions are based on tradition, scientific theories, and limited research. Although every attempt has been made to provide accurate information, neither the author nor the publishers can be held accountable for any omission or error. The author and the publisher specifically disclaim any liability that is incurred from the use or the application of the contents of this book. This information is provided for general educational purposes only and is not intended to constitute (i) medical advice or counseling; (ii) the practice of medicine, including psychiatry, psychology, psychotherapy, or the provision of health care diagnosis or treatment; (iii) the creation of a physician/patient or clinical relationship; or (iv) an endorsement, recommendation, or sponsorship of any third-party product or service by the author or the author's affiliates, agents, employees, consultants, or service providers. If you have or suspect that you have a medical problem, contact your health care provider right away.

Preface

There is an unparalleled Joy that you can only truly experience when your heart is free from worry and attachment to outcomes, appearance, and influence, which the inner critic constantly uses to keep you safe by habitually reminding you of your failures and mistakes rather than your triumphs.

But you've got bills to pay, a job to keep, decisions to make, investments to monitor, kids to raise, pets to care for, goals, dreams, passions, a need to push forward, a need to hold back, an identity to uphold, an image to keep, places to be, things to do, people to see—the Spector of time's passage is always looming.

It will get done, it will all get done...take a deep breath and know that it will all get done.

There's so much energy in that description, so much struggle, so much angst, anxiety, and fear percolating underneath all of those experiences. That energy is something we've come to ignore or dismiss. To a certain extent, it's so much a part of us that we're somewhat addicted and can't imagine life without it. We believe its presence is necessary to keep us moving along the right path. That energy is what we are going to learn to address productively together, instead of ignoring it passively.

This book is dedicated to it all happening for you and getting through it all without losing yourself.

Solutions (instinct and intuition can only be present in moments of clarity) cannot be truly clear with all of that pressure. You cannot find Joy when you are under stress!

Introduction

This is a book about *You*.

At this moment, you are probably thinking, "Wait a minute, who is *she*? She doesn't know a thing about me!" Yes, I do.

No matter how many hours you fill in your day, you can always use more time. You're generally quite focused, yet your mind drifts back and forth all day over things you need to do, should do, want to do—*didn't do*—all while you're in the midst of doing something else. It's hard to stay in the present moment. You enjoy your friends but really don't get as much time with them as you'd like. This includes your sex life, which also gets crammed in there with everything else. *Free time?* Does the extra 15 minutes that you spend in the bathroom count (after you've taken care of everything and everybody else)? *Food?* Well, let's just say you've promised to do better, but that too gets buried with other good intentions, such as getting more sleep. Sleep? Oh, yeah. It's that thing you do in between doing all that other stuff. There is a lot of time spent *doing*, yet nothing ever feels quite done.

How did I know all that about you? We all get so isolated and caught up in that tornado of thoughts between our ears that we don't realize everyone else around us is dealing with the same stuff—to a lesser or greater degree—and we're forced to wear these masks to show the world that we have everything under control. Your experience is not unique and you are not alone—it just seems that way. So in your isolation you feel overwhelmed, or like somewhat of a fraud or failure, or two seconds from a major cataclysmic event. Yet, you keep juggling all the balls in the air and you keep doing what needs to be done. You're frustrated and exhausted—*and so is everyone around you!* STRESS!

We're going to change that, you and I. None of us are immune from the highs and lows, the victories and the trials of human experience. No matter how careful you are, no matter how you attempt to control your attractions and ambitions, no matter how attentively you try to employ only positive thoughts, no matter how hard you try *not* to make mistakes, they will happen. Recognize that these are just transitions. KNOW this. They will not last. When we face an issue, we *change* it. Slow down to experience and acknowledge the emotions inherent in that moment and then *get moving!* It's not a dead end. There's no point in staying there. Do not define your *self* by periods of transition.

Grief and loss are particularly compounded emotional events. Ultimately, you must appreciate that the departed would want you to continue your life in Joy and Love. It's not fair to use their passing as an excuse for you to give up or give in to destructive behaviors.

Please note that I did not mention the concepts of "forgiveness" or "seeking closure." Wherever possible, these are wonderful, and can even happen spontaneously in time. But these can be both elusive and unnecessarily burdensome in other instances. Alexander Pope once said, "To err is human, to forgive, Divine." Is it not possible that he was alluding to the fact that some transgressions go well beyond the mere mortal capacity for the level of comprehension and compassion necessary for forgiveness? In those situations, to load yourself with such an irrational expectation will only slow you down on your path, but move on we must, for it is what we humans do. Having moved out of Africa and across the globe, we continued to move out to the stars. Change and movement are necessary for our survival. Occasionally, you must move forward without the Grace of forgiveness or closure.

Sometimes, a particularly negative part of your past must be identified as "just a past experience"; send a flow of love back to your past self for having lived through it, and now let go of it. It's not easy, but that is not where you are today. Now. Respect the emotional vibration of it—don't resist—and then let it out of your system. Letting go is neither defeat, acceptance, nor turning your back on it. Again, don't let it define who you are.

Letting go may not happen all at once. Aspects of a memory may return and once again you must recognize and release. A memory is just a memory. A thought is just a thought. Your memories and thoughts are *not your life*. You get to create and recreate your life in each moment by the thoughts that you choose.

Anytime you feel "negative emotion" (fear, doubt, worry, anger) slow down and recognize that there's something to learn there. *Otherwise*, you would not be feeling this. In all situations, your response will determine whether a crisis is intensified or reduced, or whether another person is honored or diminished. Turn inward and ask yourself, "What is it that I really want here?" And without further judgment or admonishment, simply turn your attention to what you *do* want and to what you would prefer to feel, and move forward from that point. Liken it to a car skidding or spinning out of control. You need to keep your eyes on where you want to be and continue to steer toward it. Getting to consistent happiness happens for you when you habitually access thoughts that empower you and let go of those that do not. It takes practice, just like any other skill. You can be happy in any moment when you choose to tap into it.

You can choose to learn a lesson before waving goodbye to the past, but not one used as a stick to whack yourself with. You have been tested and *you're still here*. Ask yourself what you want out of this life *now*! Use that past only to identify what it is that you really *do* want in life (what really engages you, brings you joy). Take a look at what you already have in order to decide what's worthy of keeping and what really doesn't deserve any more of your time. It's *your* time and we're going to reclaim it. We're also going to reclaim your Joy while we're at it.

Right now, in this moment, there is nothing that you need to conquer or overcome, no inadequacy to apologize for, no failure to cling to and regret. That was in your past; as of today, you can let all of that go.

That pain serves absolutely no purpose except to weigh you down and keep you from your Joy.

At the very core, the essence of your being, you were designed for Joy. Want proof? Every single living thing moves instinctively away from the flames of fire, knowing the pain and destruction it will bring. You too move intuitively away from that which brings pain. Only when we're out of balance does this natural proclivity alter. (STRESS!) So make no mistake: *You* are a complex jumble of fabulousness, and the collection of experiences that make up your life is amazing!

Joy, like Love, is not a right to be challenged, not something that you earn or buy, not a prize you win—and it cannot be lost or found...it simply is. Someone you're with may heighten this awareness and vibration in you, but it was already there. It's always there. Although Love is considered an emotion, I'd campaign strongly that it is a vital nutrient, every bit as important as the air we breathe or water we drink. This makes self-love all the more important as a life skill. We're going to tune into that more often from now on. In each moment, each of us can make choices to bring us back to our natural state of Joy, Love, and well-being. Again, like any skill, it takes practice and patience. We're going to do more of that.

Now you'll wonder, "What if the people around me don't go along and accept these changes that I make to build a new, lighter, happier, more fulfilled me?" You not only have the right to create positive change in your life, you have the obligation. Through inaction, you will sooner or later find yourself running head-long into the brick wall of your stubborn resolve, your "need to please," or your indifference. As author Ayn Rand said, "We can ignore reality, but we can't ignore the consequences of ignoring reality." These traits have been shown to cause dis-ease. Your thoughts, attitudes, friendships, and associations have enormous influence over your health (as we'll explore together in the first chapter).

Any resistance or conflict that separates you from your Joy must be severely limited or completely eliminated. Harsh, but necessary. Feeling happy, healthy, and a sense of harmony and well-being is not a selfish act. Your happiness is the most significant contribution that you can make.

When you do this, you become a catalyst for everyone around you; every object of your attention benefits when you feel good.

While you're at it, resist picking at what you perceive in others as their faults, lacks, and shortfalls. Life is a mirror and we find only ourselves reflected in those around us. Consider what your judgment may teach you about yourself. Everyone does not need to hear or share your opinion, and your opinions may change as you gain more experience and tools. You cannot know where someone else is on their road—drive *your* car.

Let's change our focus and use a Shakespeare quote as our starting point: "To be, or not to be."

Now we're going to have more time to "be more, stress less." This simple shift will make every single thing that you do simpler, higher quality, and ultimately bring you a feeling of more satisfaction and Joy. You will be more aware, alive, and finally catch up to that tail you keep chasing. We're going to change the way that you experience your experience.

Another thing that you'll see quite clearly is how focusing on Being will help you move quite easily toward optimal physical and mental health as well. All from Being more and stressing less!

1

What is in your environment?
Who is in your environment?
Where is your environment?
How are you feeling in your body?

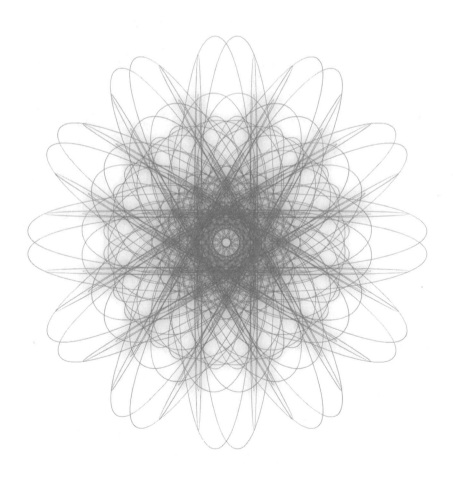

What Makes Us Sick?

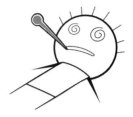

For decades, science and doctors frightened us with scary warnings about predisposition to cancers and other illness (or "genetic determinism") that could be inherited from our family members. But more current, accurate research has proven that our genes aren't in the driver's seat.

Through epigenetics, we now know it's our environment that is in control—your genetic make-up is just a tiny fraction of the equation that determines your health. Your environment is more than just the air, soil, water, and climate. It's the complete combination of your diet, lifestyle, community, and cultural conditions that influence your life. These can and *do* change the expression of your genes.

We now understand that even your thoughts are another extremely important factor, from reactions to stress to your beliefs about the possibility of becoming sick.

You can learn a lot more information about epigenetics in Dr. Bruce Lipton's book *The Biology of Belief*, which says that we all perceive or make little judgments about our environment and then our biology adjusts to the information (or signals) that we send it about what we're experiencing—whether we are happy, aroused, sad, frightened, or under stress. This happens even when our perception is *wrong*.[1] If I suggest that you imagine a rich, delicious candy bar sitting in your coat pocket, your body, solely upon my suggestion, will begin making changes in blood sugar levels in anticipation of the tasty treat.

Misperceptions about health and healing can accumulate throughout your lifetime with simple childhood associations, family superstitions, urban myths, or inaccurate news reporting. We also acquire limiting, self-sabotaging habitual thought patterns (worry, fear, doubt, anger), attitudes, and beliefs that chip away at our strength, health, and vitality.

Even if you're just working under misperceptions of your environment due to an inaccurate judgment, faulty understanding, or increased sensitivity, imbalance to your biology will occur. This explains why even young healthy people with no family history of disease can end up with cancer or some other ailment. There are even reports of healthy children adopted into a family with cancer history who develop that specific cancer. In all of these cases, their bodies have reacted to something in their environment.

Biology 101: Your DNA is the blueprint that informs the proteins that make up life. DNA is made up of two unique sequenced helical chains. One side of this chain is a physical compliment of the other, meaning the two strands are mirror images of each other. DNA is responsible for copying and replicating itself (RNA).

You're not just a single entity. Your body is a collection of more than 50 trillion cells and in one year you replace a whopping 98 percent of ALL the cells in your body. For every one cell of "you" there are 10 bacterial cells hitching a ride. You are actually a walking, talking, breathing colony of ever-changing and adapting cells.

Inside each cell, the chromosome will have two helical strands. Each of those strands will make a replication of itself and create two chromosomes—one will go into one daughter cell and the other will go into the other daughter cell. Simple, *right?*

The cell membrane—that thin little wall—is actually a functional element. Once it was thought just to be an irrelevant barrier, the skin that separates two dynamic realms, the inside and the outside of this ever-changing cellular universe. But really that thin cell membrane reads the conditions or environmental signals that your body sends it in reaction to some stimuli you've experienced, and then it actively adjusts, allowing or denying chemical messengers access to come and go. So although earlier science taught us that the nucleus was important, it's actually just taking orders from the membrane. The membrane acts quite simply as the "brain" of your cell and it takes its orders from you, or, more importantly, *your reaction to your environment.*

For a century, science incorrectly taught us that occasionally an error occurs within the billions of copied code chains, creating a change in the amino acids and therefore causing a protein with an altered structure (or mutation). These were named "Spontaneous Random Mutations" and they were given sole responsibility for all kinds of evolution and disease.

Well, it's *completely wrong!* Research biologists have discovered "repair mechanisms" right within our cell nuclei. These specialized proteins' sole function is to repair any errors, making it far less likely that all the events that led to evolution were caused by random process, because there was a very efficient mechanism in place to maintain fidelity.

Now why is that so darned important? Because you were not randomly created! Before this recent understanding, science made it seem as though your biology changed based on mistakes—crazy chance happenings that your body developed any ol' way. Instead, human biology changed in direct response to the environment around us. It kept us safe by adapting to environmental changes.

Based on this evidence, an experiment conducted by Dr. John Cairns, reported in the 1988 *British Journal of Nature*, proved that when an organism is stressed in reaction to its environment, it responds by that cell creating an enzyme (protein) to induce a mutation within the chromosome—*purposely*.[2] When we're under stress, we have elevated levels of malondialdehyde (MDA), a product that stems from the oxidation of fatty acids and that degrades the integrity of your cells. More studies, such as the research conducted by F. Marotta in 2011, concluded that *psychosocial stress* can cause system-wide imbalance of cellular homeostasis, accompanied by elevated oxidative stress and pro-inflammatory activity.[3] This is proof that genetic mutation, evolution, or alteration is in direct response to environment.

So why is that significant? Why have I dragged you all the way back to your seventh-grade science class? Because this now puts extreme emphasis on the absolute need for you to create a more balanced environment for yourself—one that includes nurturing, a bonding emotional partnership, supportive friendships, an engaging work environment, fundamental quality nutrition, clean water, rest, and external and internal balance. So ask yourself these questions:

» **What** is in your environment?

» **Who** is in your environment?

» **Where** is your environment?

» **How** are you feeling in your body?

Answers to these questions weigh far more heavily on your health than the chains of proteins that you're made from. Even the Center for Disease Control (CDC) states that 85 percent of disease is caused by emotions.[4] It is likely that this factor may be more important than all the other physical aspects combined. So shouldn't we make attention to our emotional changes a priority?

Take a moment and simply think of your brain as a digital device and disease as one of its programs, which is switched on in specific circumstances of high stress or conflict, and switches off when the high or prolonged stress or conflict is released or resolved!

The signals that control your biology come from your body's direct response to your environment, which then creates the chemical reactions that cause illness, or health and well-being. It's the environment and how you perceive it and react to it, that is, psychological factors, that make all the difference in your health.

Even the greatest minds in quantum mechanics have not succeeded in overriding the effects of perception. The very nature of matter is expressed as "wave-particle duality," the concept that all energy (and therefore all matter) exhibits both wave-like and particle-like properties depending on how it is perceived.

"The field is the sole governing agency of the particle," is a quote commonly attributed to Einstein. Biologically speaking, we are those particles. Life, as we are able to comprehend it, is a simple collection of tinker toy–like chains of proteins, or at least that's how we make the distinction within the limitations of science.

Signals bind to proteins and change their shape; those shape-changes provide for the behavior in human physiology. Signal + Protein = Behavior. Signals come from your environment, or more specifically, your *reaction* to your environment. Energetic signals would be what we call "thoughts," and therefore, these too have significant effect!

What about that second element called protein? Could protein be the cause of disease? Well, a protein itself is based on the sequence of amino acids and may in fact be defective (mutated or distorted DNA or genetics). But that is very, *very* rare. It affects fewer than 5 percent of the people on this planet. With a percentage so small in contrast to the percentage of people actually exhibiting disease or cancer, the overwhelming conclusion is that the majority of illness and disease is caused by something in the signal, that is, the environment—not the protein.

What in your environment can cause a signal that interferes with protein function?

» **Trauma:** Some kind of major accident that results in a distortion of the info being exchanged between your brain and your body's cells, tissues, and organs. One example would be a broken limb that heals improperly, thereby physically impeding the transmission of the nervous system's signal.

» **Toxicity:** We've filled our environment with a wide variety of toxins. These can garble the signal's information on its path between your nervous system and your cells and tissues.

» **Reaction to the Environment:** By far the most common reason. Yep, the actions of your mind—perceptions, beliefs, and attitudes—including STRESS. Your health relies completely on your nervous system's ability to correctly distinguish information from your environment and appropriately adapt life-sustaining behaviors. If your mind misinterprets environmental signals and generates an inappropriate response, survival is threatened because the body's behaviors become out of synch with the environment.

The genes that you inherited from Mom and Dad are no more than blueprints. They are not self-actualizing or even controlling devices. Their fate is determined by information from your environment. You know this from your own experience. Ten people may be exposed to cold germs in an office; some will catch the cold, and each of those people will all have varying levels of symptoms. Others may not catch it at all. What's different? The strength of their immune systems, which is based on diet, sleep, fitness, relationships, and mood (including how stressed they feel).

This is not to say that stress in your environment is pure evil. Let's face it: some stress is absolutely necessary and appropriate. If early man had not kept alert and appropriately fearful of saber-toothed tigers, we would not be here to stress over food prices. Remember, perception is key and determines whether or not the stress is continual. Small amounts of stress have even been found to start the redistribution of immune cells, which can possibly aid your survival by sending protection where stress is occurring.

However, the major point is learning to monitor how you perceive the stress in your environment. That is why, in Chapter 2, we're going to learn how to stop for just a few minutes and take stock. We tend to glance right by our stress and stressors. This multi-level denial allows your body's stress reactions to accumulate and build up. At that point, it is more difficult to get it under control and even small things will set off a reaction that is out of proportion with your normal day-to-day feelings.

Research has proven that in those stress-filled moments, defining your stress as enhancing or as debilitating will determine not only how your body reacts, but how quickly your biological responses subside.

Through using the techniques described in this book, you can, in time, learn to use your stress and make it work for you instead of against you. You can positively alter your behavioral and physiological outcomes from stress in your environment through learning to change your reaction. So, what makes us sick? We can answer that with another question.

What's in Your Environment?

Here are a couple common things you can consider in your physical environment to get the ball rolling:

» Reduce your exposure to environmental toxins such as pesticides, household chemical cleaners, Teflon and Teflon-coated fabrics, plastics with Bisphenol A (BPA), fluorinated telomeres in fast-food packaging, dry-cleaning chemicals, synthetic air fresheners, and air pollution.

» When possible, limit your exposure and provide protection for yourself from radiation produced by large utility poles and transformer station groups, cell phone towers, base stations, and WiFi stations.

That's just a start. There are many more things to consider, which are personal and more specific to your life. Ask yourself: What do you control in your environment that you can change, balance, or improve to increase your health right now?

2

What's affectionately referred to as "Belly Fat"
is a direct indicator of STRESS!

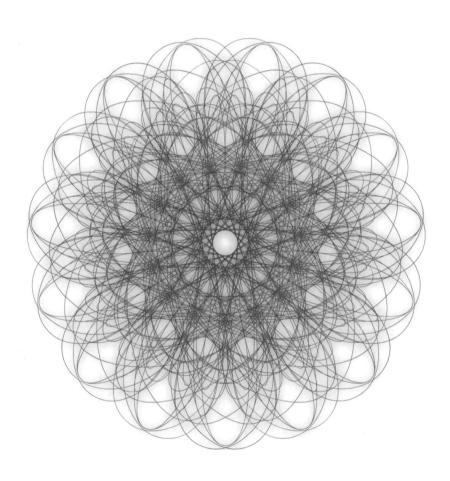

Stress: The Equal Opportunity Assassin

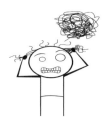

Why do I keep harping on the need to let things go? Or the need to Be more and stress less? Because stress will kill you. We all walk around talking about how stressed out we are as part of casual conversation, but it is a serious concern. It affects all socio-economic levels, geographic areas, age groups, genders, and races. They've got it in China, Turkey, and Iceland. It is so pervasive that the United States has named April National Stress Awareness month![1]

Chronic stress can cause issues such as suppression of thyroid function, cognitive impairment, increased blood pressure, decreased bone density, blood sugar imbalances, fatigue and weakness, suppression of the immune system, muscle and bone loss, moodiness or depression, hormonal imbalances, skin problems, hair loss, autoimmune disorders, and insulin resistance.

Another statistic related to too much stress is heart attacks. In the United States, a heart attack occurs about every 20 seconds, with a heart attack death about every minute. The CDC estimates that 25.6 million, or 11.3 percent of all people aged 20 years or older in the United States have diabetes.[2] Here is a list of life's most stressful events:

- » Death of your spouse, family member, or friend.
- » Divorce or marital separation.
- » Personal injury or illness.
- » Marriage.
- » Losing your job.
- » Retirement.
- » Drastic change in the health of a family member.
- » Pregnancy.
- » Sexual dysfunction.
- » Birth of a child.
- » Change in business status.

» Change in financial status.

» Unresolved relationship problems.

You see, stress is a relatively new phenomenon on the human development timeline. Our bodies have not had a chance to adapt to this new concept. When your nervous system gets an intense jolt of stress, your body reacts in the same way that it would if you were in eminent danger of death.

Say you're on the phone with customer service and you've been transferred about three or four times while waiting to speak to a real person. You're pretty steamed, and the obnoxious music playing is only adding to your irritation. You reach for something to munch on as you pass the time. FINALLY! Someone comes on the line, but the call gets dropped.

Let's take a look at what just happened in your body during that episode. Your nervous system has alerted your brain that there is massive danger—possibly a man-eating tiger. Your brain gets the signal and snaps into action. Sometimes this is called the "fight-or-flight response." The adrenal glands, two walnut-sized, innocent-looking triangular-shaped organs that sit perched atop your kidneys, are switched on. They start releasing stress hormones through the synthesis of corticosteroids (cortisol and catecholamines such as epinephrine [adrenaline] and norepinephrine). The cortisol releases glucose into your bloodstream for energy. In other words, your blood sugar gets immediately elevated under stress. You can't fight danger when your blood sugar is low, so it amps up to help you meet the challenge.

A domino effect takes place. All available resources have been switched over to increase your energy level toward movement, because it's assumed that you're about to sprint away full speed from danger and your brain wants you to have every ounce of strength it can muster for your mad dash. So it minimizes all the resources that were going to your digestion (after all, you aren't going to have time for fine dining while on the run), and it reduces your carbohydrate, protein, and fat metabolism, as well as fluid and electrolyte balance. It lowers your immunity and inflammatory responses. Muscle tissue is tapped to produce more glucose for energy. Triglycerides get mobilized from your fat tissues. You actually have reduced sensitivity to pain and your skin temperature changes. It even turns off your sex drive. (This is no time for making "whoopie.") And the little guys in the boiler room are working overtime to pump up your cardiovascular function, speeding up the heart and contracting blood vessels, which increases your blood pressure. Adjustments are made in the resistance to airflow both in and out of your lungs by altering the diameter of the branches of the bronchial tree. Meanwhile, it calculates your likely need for quick-burning energy to get you going (glucose and triglycerides were already consumed by your cells in preparation for activity), so that subliminal craving you had to munch on something sweet or fatty was not random. That was your brain nudging you to provide it with some additional kindling for this fire it is building. You're irritated talking on the phone, but your body now has the boiler fully stoked and blazing hot. *Whew!* A lot happens very quickly when you are under stress.

The phone call ends. You turn your attention to other matters. What's your body going to do now with all of that extra energy and resources? You're not giving it a way to burn it off because you're still sitting there; you didn't take the sprint your body anticipated after all. The only option left is to store it, but where should it be stored? Somewhere with easy access just in case the man-eating tiger comes back. How about…*your abdomen*!

Yep! What's affectionately referred to as "belly fat" is a direct indicator of STRESS! Belly fat is associated with many health problems, including cardiovascular diseases, asthma, sleep apnea, diabetes, stroke, high cholesterol, and joint diseases. Why? Prolonged or high levels of cortisol, that is, stress, takes all of your body's natural defense mechanisms offline.

Cortisol Out-of-Control

On one hand, too much cortisol severely weakens your immune system by inhibiting the very necessary production of white blood cells that protect your body against foreign invaders, more specifically lymph node and lymphocyte function. This sets into motion increased susceptibility to infections and cancer. On the other hand, too little cortisol leads to an overactive immune system and autoimmune disease. What's left is very reduced functionality, and even that's compromised by the crappy nutrition you're giving your body, along with lack of sleep, little exercise, and all the shallow breathing you do. Your body can't even get rid of the truckload of toxins it's routinely exposed to, much less this extra stress.

Stress is as harmful to the immune systems of children as it is to the adults stressing out around them. A 2014 study conducted by a research group at Jönköping University in Sweden, published in the American periodical *Journal of Immunology*, demonstrated this clearly.[3] The study included 5-year-old children from families reporting typical high stress difficulties, such as divorce or unemployment. Their results showed unmistakably that children in highly stressed families had high cortisol levels, which is a biological marker for stress. The research study supported the fact that a high level of stress negatively affects immune system function because it fundamentally loses resistance when your body is under this condition. Instead, your immune system will react to substances in the body that should be left alone, which perhaps is linked to an autoimmune reaction.

Did I rudely mention the weight you're putting on? Consistent, prolonged stress and the overproduction of cortisol play a direct role in your "comfort" food cravings, overeating, fatigue, and storing excess body fat. Serotonin release is triggered by a carbohydrate load (sugar and so on). Serotonin is a chemical that helps you to maintain a "happy feeling," and seems to assist in keeping moods under control by aiding sleep, calming anxiety, and relieving depression. There are many who feel that eating carbs when we're under stress is really an unconscious attempt to invoke this feel-good serotonin release, in addition to the quick energy that they bring.

Another aspect of the cortisol release produced by chronic stress is that it causes bone cells to stop growing or to release calcium into the bloodstream. This is why excessive cortisol levels can lead to osteoporosis.

Stress is also a factor in cancer. For example, studies proved that stress can promote breast cancer cell colonization of bone. They showed that activation of the sympathetic nervous system—your fight-or-flight response to stress—sets up the bone environment for breast cancer cell metastasis. Metastasis is defined as the spread of cancer cells to distant organs and bones. It is more likely to lead to the death of patients than the primary breast tumor, said Florent Elefteriou, PhD, director of the Vanderbilt Center for Bone Biology. "Preventing metastasis is really the goal we want to achieve," he continued. "Efforts to reduce stress and depression in patients with cancer may have unappreciated benefits in terms of metastasis prevention."[4]

O My Omentum!

Biology 101: You've got three kinds of fat: fat in your bloodstream (triglycerides), subcutaneous fat (which lies just beneath the surface of your skin), and your omentum fat (visceral).

Your omentum is a fatty layer of tissue that hangs off the middle of your colon and drapes over the intestines inside your abdomen. If you've ever heard of visceral fat or intra-abdominal adiposity (IAA), this is just another way of describing the omentum.

It is split into two segments called the greater and lesser omentum. For some reason, they didn't show you this in your high school textbook, did they? The "greater," is a mass that sits in front of the stomach and the "lesser" covers your liver. Both share a singular objective, which is to store fat. When the greater omentum is especially large, the abdomen may appear stiff and distended. You may have seen a person who is not considerably overweight, but they might show definite signs of a significantly large omentum. The location of your omentum, so close to your vital organs, makes it their best source for energy, which is good news, right? Well, not exactly.

Ever wonder what your body does with the constant barrage of daily toxins that it doesn't process (like hydrogenated oils and trans-fats)? Your body stores them away in your fat tissue. So this fat released from your omentum also happens to rapidly and constantly travel to your liver and vital organs, carrying along with it its increased levels of toxic substances.

This processed material is then shipped off to your arteries, where it ends up causing health risks such as high LDL (Lousy—*oops*, I mean Low Density) cholesterol. Can you see why this type of fat is so consistently linked to serious diseases?

But wait, there's more! The more omentum fat you have, the less adiponectin you produce. Adiponectin is a very important stress- and inflammation-reducing chemical related to the hunger-controlling hormone called leptin. This not only imbalances your ability to know when you are full after you have a meal, it also starts a cascade of inflammatory processes, which can lead to diabetes, high blood pressure, and hardening of the arteries.

Your omentum also receives and stores hormones like cortisol (which we just discussed). High amounts of stress stimulate its growth. Under a great deal of continual stress, you'll find that reducing the size of this organ is very problematic. You cannot simply diet, but you must reduce your stress through other therapies such as relaxation techniques and lifestyle changes, which we'll talk a lot about in this book. The bottom line is stress and belly fat are inescapably linked.

And then there's the rust…isoprostanes. It's oxygen or oxidation that causes iron to rust and silver to tarnish. A similar concept causes your cells to rust and tarnish. When you get stressed out, a serious imbalance occurs between increased exposure to free radicals (see Chapter 4) and the antioxidant defenses your body needs to address them.

The consequence is the creation of oxidative chemicals that cause accelerated aging, increased cardiovascular risk, and vulnerability to various chronic and acute illnesses, including fairly typical things such as colds. In fact, Vanderbilt University researchers discovered that accurate and uncomplicated assessments of oxidative stress inside your body could actually be determined by just the measurement of your isoprostanes level.

The Emotional Aspects of Chronic Stress

"Emotions adjust not only our mental, but also our bodily states. This way, they prepare us to react swiftly to the dangers, but also to the opportunities such as pleasurable social interactions present in the environment.

Awareness of the corresponding bodily changes may subsequently trigger the conscious emotional sensations, such as the feeling of happiness," says Aalto University assistant professor Lauri Nummenmaa.[5]

Here's a short list of the most frequently reported emotional responses to stress:

» Anxiety.
» Insomnia or difficulty falling asleep.
» Depression.
» Feeling loss of control.

Do you have enough reasons to reduce your stress levels now? Do you see the relevance and how stress plays out in every aspect of your health? You might be surprised at how reducing stress in other parts of your environment can put your whole life in perspective!

Mitigation

It starts with the concept that we opened the book with the mission of Being more and stressing less. *Acknowledge* that the stress is present in the current moment. Of course this requires that you Be in the moment and not on auto-pilot.

We are so attached to our masks that tell the world that we've got everything handled and everything's under control. This doesn't mean that you need to take out a billboard or start a blog about your stress. The whole concept of "I'm managing my stress" is bogus. You don't "manage" a raging tiger! You calm yourself and then you determine the next best course of action. This is the moment where you can greatly reduce and even reverse some of the negative physical and mental effects of stress. How you define or re-define your stress in this moment will make all the difference.

Research has shown that when you reappraise what the stress of a given situation means, you now control its effects. How do you reframe the tumult that can exist in your daily life? It starts by simply noticing what's going on in your mind, your body, your surroundings, and so on.

The Stop Technique
(Adapted from Johnny "Ananda" Norman)

The Stop Technique is an extremely simple step that will help you focus and heal, because it gives you such valuable information about where you are (and even more about what's going on around you). This technique takes about two minutes. The world *will* spin without you for a minute or two.

1. At several points during your day, STOP!
2. Wherever you are, whatever you're doing, STOP!
3. Absorb the scene around you. What's going on? Survey sights, sounds, colors, and odors.
4. Now take a single deep breath.
5. In this moment that you are taking for yourself, there is nothing else for you to think about or accomplish.
6. Focus and really draw in your awareness of your:

   » Heart rate. Really feel your pulse and notice the sensation in your chest.
   » Breathing. Is it shallow? (Is it from a stuffy nose or is it tension?)
   » Skin temperature. Are you warm? Cool? Is it dry in the room? Is the humidity high?
   » Tension. Any kinks or knots your body is holding onto? Ask yourself what the source might be; is it just a matter of shifting positions or are you stifling the impulse to choke the living daylights out of someone?

7. Relax your muscles.
8. Analyze how you feel. Are you happy, bored, hopeful, anxious, rested, frustrated, calm, intimidated, guilty, accomplished, scattered, claustrophobic, at ease? Really put a *word* to exactly what you feel in this particular moment.
9. Now what do you *want* to feel? How would you like to feel *right now?* Would you like to be on a beach somewhere relaxing or out with friends? Is joy one of the things that you'd like to feel?

Leaving behind whatever else you were doing before or must do later, in this moment conjure for yourself a feeling of warm happiness. You may need to imagine a scene or evoke a memory (although it is better if you can just reach inside and find "happy" among all the other feelings that you've catalogued in your life). Engage all of your senses and really sense the Joy rising up from somewhere inside you. Smile from ear to ear—bring out the gums—and in this moment your feeling will shift to feeling good and your body will respond.

The simple act of smiling may help to immediately reduce symptoms associated with stress and anxiety. Mark Stibich, PhD, consultant at Columbia University, believes that "If you can slow your breathing down and change your expression, you may be able to turn around the stress cascade."[6] Dr. Stibich is the author of several articles about the positive health effects of "Duchene" smiling, involving muscles in the mouth, cheeks, and eyes, which are considered "real smiles."

According to Stibich, smiling:

» Lowers blood pressure.
» Reduces stress.
» Stimulates the immune system.

The STOP Technique is simple yet *effective* and brings immediate results. Consider what you gain from this simple 2-minute exercise:

» Observation of your immediate setting brings invaluable information you may otherwise miss with your head buried in the sand. You'll pick up on things you wouldn't have noticed.
» Your heart rate slows (brings down elevated blood pressure).
» Breathing evens out (the oxygen provides energy, which means an increase in your energy level).
» Blood sugar levels can improve.
» Feelings such as frustration, anger, or fear can quickly be replaced by a focused, relaxed state of mind.
» Merely thinking of happiness releases endorphins throughout your body. (Endorphins are those feel-good, natural painkillers.)
» You are more efficient at *any* task you return to.

Like any skill, these take some practice. Repetition is your friend.

The Importance of Nature

Whenever possible, get yourself to a natural setting. Take a walk in a local park. Dr. Marc Berman and fellow researchers at the University of Michigan found that "performance on memory and attention tests improved by 20 percent after study subjects paused for a walk through an arboretum. When these people were sent on a break to stroll down a busy street in town, no cognitive boost was detected."[7]

Just to really hit the point home, University of Washington researchers found that plasma screens displaying an outdoor scene were about as effective as a blank wall in reducing test subjects' tension (as measured by a drop in heart rates).[8]

So that means you're gonna have to actually move your body outdoors if you want to benefit from nature. What's amazing is that in as little as 10 minutes, you produce biochemical reactions that increase levels of the mood chemical serotonin, helping to alleviate depression, relieve stress, and boost your daytime energy.

You begin to see clearly now that wherever your mind is, wherever your thoughts are, there you are *and there your body is*. The good news is that you can move your thoughts and your mind somewhere else with relative ease and literally within a few breaths. There is an obvious and undeniable mind-body connection when you really take notice—and that's the central point. *Take notice!*

Reappraisal and Reframing Stress

It is so important that you now take signs of stress—your arousal (agitated, quick, or looping thoughts, rapid pulse, sweaty palms, and so on)—and interpret them in a more positive light to really *use them*. That's right! Turn the energy that comes with them into something that you can use. For example, let's say you've had a challenging conversation with a work colleague or your boss that has left you agitated and stressed. Once you've done the Stop Technique and toned down your levels a little bit, tell yourself, "I'm going to use this agitation to get xyz report (or some other activity) done." You've acknowledged the energy from the stress *and* you're giving it a positive target for release. You're now *using* your stress.

Shawn Achor, an expert in positive psychology, says, "When people have a stress in their life, they can attempt to see it as a challenge, instead of a threat."[9] The shift caused by using this tool will allow the feeling of stress to be motivating rather than paralyzing.

This simple redefining technique actually causes biochemical changes. It will reduce or even reverse some of the cortisol response that we just discussed. In fact, studies suggest that moderate levels of stress enhance neural function and learning. We'll examine more techniques for this throughout the book.

As you can see, Being more and stressing less includes actively attending to your stress levels—not trying to suppress and ignore it. The more actively you take care of your stress, the better you feel, the more productive and focused you are, and ultimately the deeper your sense of satisfaction and Joy is. Be attentive.

3

Deep breathing actually signals your brain to release the hormone that invokes Joy and mood-modulation, and also helps us sleep by calming anxiety and relieving depression.

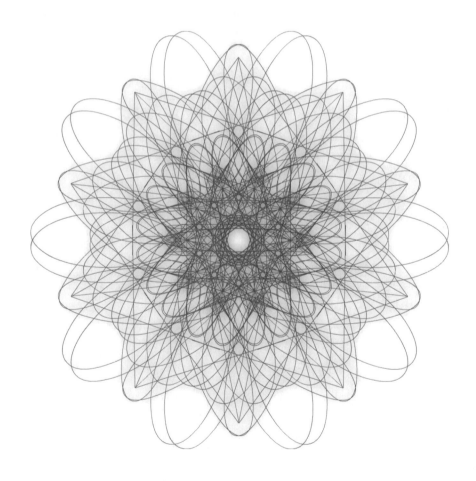

Breathe Your Way to Better Mental and Physical Health

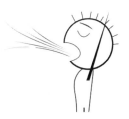

Your breath is quite literally your life force. Because approximately 90 percent of your energy is created by oxygen and nearly all of your body's actions are regulated by it, it's extremely important to get enough of it. Breathing influences every organ in your body, and as you'll learn, it also balances the brain hemispheres.

However, breathing is something that we all take for granted and are inclined to simply overlook. It is surprising how few of us actually breathe properly. Most of us are simply breathing too fast. Generally a person might have 15 to 20 breath cycles per minute, but an ideal number is 5 to 10 cycles per minute at rest. What's going on? We're all doing a lot of shallow breathing, and we need to slow it down.

Shallow breathing can often be a symptom of anxiety. Think about it for a moment. When you are frightened or stressed, you tend to hold your breath or take rapid, shallow breaths; your heart pounds and muscles clench as the adrenaline kicks in. This shallow breathing can result in fatigue and stress due to the intake of insufficient oxygen. It can also result in dizziness (due to lack of oxygen getting to your brain). However, deep breathing can flip the switch from high alert to low cruise control in a matter of seconds.

The simple act of breathing evenly and deeply through both nostrils helps you to synchronize both sides of your brain. Research has proven that your brain swaps the dominate nostril that you breathe through every 90 minutes. Your hypothalamus is responsible for the switch in nostril dominance. This subtle shift essentially controls your autonomic nervous system.

When you breathe in through the left nostril, your right brain hemisphere is stimulated. On the other hand, when you breathe in through your right nostril, your left brain hemisphere is stimulated. In fact, D.A. Werntz, a researcher conducting a study at the University of California at

San Diego School of Medicine, demonstrated that breathing through one nostril generated EEG activity in the opposite brain hemisphere.[1]

Your brain's right and left hemispheres have different functions. Generally, your left hemisphere is linked with all of your verbal, linear, rational activities, while your right hemisphere handles spatial, nonlinear, and intuitive activities. Dr. Shirley Telles, director of Research at Patanjali Yogpeeth, Haridwar, India, and head of the Indian Council of Medical Research for Advanced Research in Yoga and Neurophysiology, proved that when nostril dominance was forced to a particular side of the brain, the task performance associated with that side was actually enhanced. For example, right nostril breathing improved verbal skills associated with the left hemisphere, while left nostril breathing was shown to improve the intuitive or spatial skills associated with the right hemisphere.[2]

Another use of this technique is in changing your emotional state. Moods and emotions that are considered negative, such as anger, depression, or fear, seem to dominate in the right hemisphere of your brain. Meanwhile, the more positive emotions, such as joy and gratitude, dominate in your left brain. Here's the fun part: you can change that dominance, regardless of which side is dominant at the moment, by simply directing or even just imagining breath coming in through the opposite nostril. Let's say, for instance, that you'd like to stimulate more intuitive activity. Just the simple act of breathing in through your left nostril several times (by compressing the right nostril lightly), or even by simply imagining your breath coming through your left nostril, will help establish the new desired pattern.

Breathing also has many positive effects on your body, some obvious and others less so. Some scientists believe that breath is the doorway between your conscious and unconscious mind. It can definitely help relax and nourish specific parts of your body, give you better control over your parasympathetic and sympathetic nervous system, and has even been reported to play a large role in some extraordinary cures.

Breathing actively places us into what science calls a "kinesthetic" state, that is, a more "feeling" state. Recently, the work of Dr. Candace Pert revealed that the lower tips of our lungs actually have serotonin receptors that act as neurotransmitter and signaling mechanisms.[3] That's right! Deep breathing actually signals your brain to release the hormone that invokes Joy and mood-modulation, and also helps us sleep by calming anxiety and relieving depression.

Who'da thunk?! Deep breathing does so many amazing things, not to mention the toxins it removes, such as carbon dioxide, which is a waste product that our respiratory system produces. Carbon dioxide is poisonous to our body in high amounts and that's exactly why our bodies release it.

Breathing also serves as the pump for your lymphatic system, which is like your body's sewer system. Lymph vessels form a drainage system throughout your body. Your cells swim in an ocean of lymphatic fluid that carries away the waste of your immune system, including dead white blood cells, unused plasma protein, and toxins. There's a chain reaction when you breathe that causes an expansion and contraction of an organ called the diaphragm, which actually stimulates your lymphatic system and massages your internal organs, helping your body rid itself of toxins and leaving more room in the cells for an optimal exchange of oxygen. Wow! Ready to take that deep breath now?!

The best thing about deep breathing is that you can do it anywhere, even while you're doing others things. It helps lower stress, increase energy, aid mental clarity, and infuse every cell in your body with the most precious element for the body: oxygen. You can do it while driving, doing dishes, or mowing the lawn. If you happen to sit in front of a computer all day, do some deep breathing intermittently and the difference in your energy at the end of your day will be very noticeable.

The Basic "Belly Breath" (Diaphragmatic Breathing)

You may have become more accustomed to only feeling your chest rise and fall as you breathe, which is shallow breathing, but this is a little different. So, just to get a basic understanding of it until you can do it instinctively, sit in a comfortable position with your hands on your knees. Relax your shoulders. Breathing through your nose, inhale and let your relaxed stomach muscles drop while filling this lower area of your abdomen with air as deeply as you can (try counting slowly to five). At the bottom of your breath, pause for two counts. Now breathe out through your mouth (again, try counting to five). Close your eyes and repeat this combination 5 to 10 times.

A really immediate way to experience diaphragmatic or belly breathing is to simply lie on your back and breathe; your body will do it automatically from this position.

What's happening? Your lungs don't actually have a muscle of their own. Lungs are just like two loose empty bags—they cannot pull air in on their own. It's the movement of your diaphragm that draws air in and out of your body. The diaphragm is a large muscle that divides the rib cage (and its organs) from your abdominal cavity. Your diaphragm works like a bellows. As your diaphragm moves down from the base of the ribs, air is drawn through the nostrils, through the trachea and bronchial tubes, and into the many small sacs linking your lungs. As air is drawing into the lungs, they expand as they fill, simultaneously expanding your rib cage, and lifting the surface of your abdomen upward.

A more controlled and conscious movement of the diaphragm draws air more deeply into the lungs.

Forced Alternate Nostril Breathing (Pranayama—Naadi Shodhana)

This is going to knock your socks off! It is so simple and so easy to do, just 3 to 5 minutes, twice a day.

- » Sit in a comfortable position with your hands on your knees. Relax.
- » Place your right thumb on the right side of your nose, in the small groove where the nostril flares.
- » *Gently* press the right nostril closed with the right thumb.
- » *Gently* exhale through the left nostril.
- » Inhale through the left nostril.
- » Close the left nostril with your right ring finger, release your thumb, and exhale thru the right nostril.
- » Inhale through the right nostril.

» Close the right nostril with the thumb, exhale left nostril.

Continue with this rhythmic breathing, slowly and smoothly, inhaling fully, exhaling completely. Relax.

It has been proven that there is a direct connection between the *prana* or "energy" of breathing, and its influence on the actual energy levels that you experience in your body. For example, cellular metabolism (reactions in your cells to produce energy) is regulated by the oxygen provided during your breathing. The purpose of breath training is not to override your body's autonomic systems, even though there is strong evidence that pranayama breathing techniques effect oxygen consumption and metabolism.

The effects of 10 minutes of forced alternate nostril breathing (FANB) were studied with 18 trained subjects and measured using an EEG. One group of FANB used left nostril inhaling and right nostril exhaling, while the other used just the opposite (right nostril inhaling and left nostril exhaling).

So what did the results show? The average power in their brain wave patterns actually increased during FANB with both types of nostril breathing. There was a definite rise in the strength of their overall brain wave pattern energy.[4]

In addition, the asymmetry or unevenness of the brain hemispheres that had shown up in readings when they began the experiment decreased by the end, suggesting that FANB has a balancing effect on the functional activity of the left and right hemisphere.[5] Amazing!

Adding FANB to your daily routine is a giant leap for you toward Being more and stressing less. Again, you will need to do this for 3 to 5 minutes, twice a day, but that small amount will bring wonderful benefits to your body and mind. In the process, you get a reduction in stress and blood pressure, strengthening of abdominal and intestinal muscles, and relief of general body aches and pains. At the same time you're also promoting better blood flow, releasing harmful toxins from the body, and improving sleep. All of these benefits will result in an increased energy level.

Getting out of the way, relaxing, and letting things flow will help allow healing to happen; it's a natural experience that your body wants. When everything is flowing, you are healthy and vital.

Breathe, deeply and often.

4

"Let food be thy medicine and medicine be thy food."
—Hippocrates

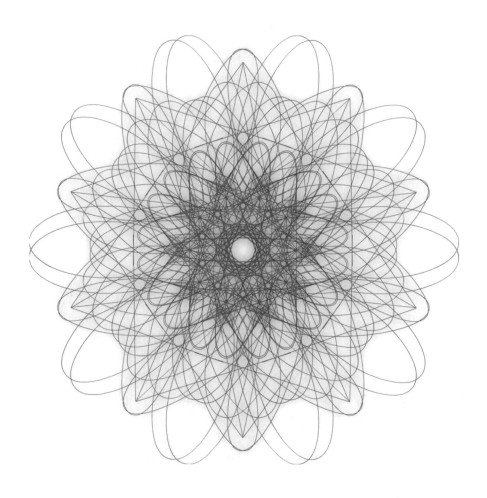

Eat, Drink, and Be Healthy (Food as Information)

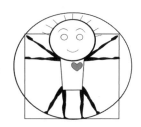

Each individual body is different. Our bodies didn't come with instruction manuals, but they do give us clues and valuable information about what they need. But how do you figure out what your body needs?

Be aware when you eat. Don't just shove food in your mouth and swallow! Take your time; really taste, savor, and enjoy your food! *This is your time*. In fact, don't "eat,"—*dine*. Find a way to make an occasion out of your mealtime and slow down. This is another area where Being more and stressing less comes into play. Your emotional state as you're eating will directly affect the way your body cells utilize the information (chemicals and energy) in your food.

Begin each meal with three deep breaths. Just stop yourself for that moment and breathe. It's so simple, but it will have a major impact. You're probably thinking, *I barely have time to eat, much less stop and breathe*, but that's the point. Slow things down; your body will thank you for it with improved digestion.

This goes for families too. Yes, it's already hard enough to get everyone to sit down together for a meal, but you're teaching them habits for a lifetime. *A lifetime*. So wrangle them in as often as possible to sit down for a meal and tell them, "We are going to have a moment of silence and take three deep breaths before we eat." It's something new—so of course you may get protests, wiggling, giggling—but eventually it will become just a part of their routine—simple habits—like reaching for your hand as they approach a street corner or brushing teeth before bed. Before you start eating, explain to them that you are going to have a moment of silence and take three deep breaths before you eat. It's something new, so of course you may get protests, wiggling, and giggling, but eventually it will become just a part of their routine.

Also consider when you might be eating for emotional reasons. Did someone tick you off and you reached for chocolate? Did your mother call and suddenly you got a craving for a pastry or comfort food? So many people self-medicate with food. It's used to fend off loneliness, depression, anger, frustration, and *STRESS*. Stop and think, then make better choices. Learn to fuel your body for optimal energy, fitness, and health!

Try as often as possible to balance the food on your plate. Let's compare carbohydrates (fast energy) to putting gasoline in your car. Proteins are your breaks—they slow down the carbs you consume so you're not hungry again as quickly! A good protein portion size is about the size of your fist. It's about the same for your carbohydrates. You will want to have a protein, carb, and something raw or green on your plate at every meal.

Any meal or snack that is high in carbohydrates will also generate a rapid rise in your blood glucose. To adjust for this rapid rise, your pancreas will secrete insulin into your bloodstream, which quickly lowers your levels of blood glucose. Why is that a bad thing? Because insulin is essentially a "storage" hormone. Early on, your body evolved insulin as a way to store excess carbohydrate calories in the form of fat, *just in case* there were times of famine. So, the insulin that's stimulated by excess carbohydrates aggressively stimulates your accumulation of body fat. Not good.

Each time you eat too much sugar, fructose, bread, pasta, or a grain product, your body gets the hormonal message (via insulin), "Hey, store more fat." This is a great benefit for certain parts of the world or during periods when calories are very scarce, but it is part of the cause of the United States obesity epidemic.

When you begin to eat more consciously and more deliberately, you'll be able to more easily sense when you are full. Gradually reduce your portion sizes. We live in a super-sized food society. Remember that you do not have to clean your plate.

Now, check for reactions. This requires a little more of that mindfulness we discussed. How does your body feel during the next few hours? Are you sluggish? Are you energized but then have a downward energy spiral, or are you fairly even in your mood and energy levels? Now you're learning what fuel (food) your body best responds to.

Please be aware that stressors in your diet—fats and hidden food allergens, the sugar you eat, high doses of the wrong oils, lack of exercise, and chronic stress—all trigger a raging, unseen chronic inflammation deep in your cells and tissues.

What's Inflammation?

Inflammation is your body's natural response to injury. Think of a time when you've had an injury, such as a cut, scrape, burn, or sprain. You know that swelling, redness, and feverish sensation that happens in the tissue surrounding it? This is a short-term heightened immune response that your body initiates in cases of trauma, infection, and allergy. Its goal is to identify the infectious or dangerous substance, then determine which cells are "self" cells (non-threatening) and which are "non-self" cells (threatening), assess the level of the threat, and finally begin a healing response to repair any resulting damage. *Great, right?*

Yep, it's all good until this response is not completely turned off. Now you've got excess immune cells that are continuously activated and disrupting other body systems. This in turn now damages healthy areas in your body, such as blood vessel linings (as in atherosclerosis), pancreatic tissue (in diabetes), joint tissue (in arthritis), and gut mucosa (in lactose and gluten intolerance). This type of inflammation is often the major cause of fluid retention, obesity, fatigue, brain fog, irritable bowel syndrome, mood problems, headaches, sinus/nasal congestion, joint pains, acne, eczema, and the list goes on. In fact, chronic inflammation leads to every one of the major chronic diseases of aging: heart disease, Type-2 diabetes, dementia, cancer, and so on.

What Causes Chronic Inflammation?

STRESS! This includes stressors from toxins in your surrounding environment, food toxins, and yes, toxic relationships. All of these can cause your body's alert system to go into hyperdrive.

Stress has now been linked directly to the onset of Type-2 diabetes. This was the finding of a ground-breaking, 35-year prospective follow-up study of 7,500 men done by the University of Gothenburg in Sweden.

How did they define stress for the study? They used the same factors that you encounter every day: irritation, anxiety, and difficulties in sleeping related to conditions at work or at home. At baseline, 15.5 percent of the men reported permanent stress related to conditions at work or home, either during the past year or during the past five years.

The results? Men who reported permanent stress had a 45 percent higher risk of developing Type-2 diabetes than those who reported to have no stress or periodic stress. This direct link between stress and diabetes was still statistically significant, even after adjusting for age, socioeconomic status, physical inactivity, BMI, systolic blood pressure, and use of blood pressure–lowering medication. "Today, stress is not recognized as a preventable cause of diabetes," says researcher Masuma Novak, leader of the study. "As our study shows that there is an independent link between permanent stress and the risk of developing diabetes, which underlines the importance of preventive measure."[1]

Stress causes inflammation. Getting a handle on stressors causing inflammation through your diet is a huge part of resolving even mental and emotional stress and the effects of external stressors from your environment, so let's take a look at the foods you eat.

There are certain foods that have been shown to cause inflammation more often. They are:

» Gluten (wheat, barley, rye, spelt, kamut).
» Oats.
» Dairy (milk, cheese, butter, yogurt).
» Corn.
» Eggs.
» Soy (tofu, soy nut butters, soy milk, soy ice cream, soy cheese, soy flour, textured soy protein (TSP), texturized vegetable protein (TVP), atsuage, aburage, soybean oil, and yuba.
» Nuts.
» Nightshade vegetables (tomatoes, potatoes, eggplant, bell peppers, tomatillos, pimento, paprika, and cayenne pepper).
» Citrus (lemons, tangerines, oranges, mandarins, grapefruits, tangelos, pummelo, kumquats, and limes).

» Yeast (baker's yeast [pizza dough, bread, doughnuts, most sour-dough bread], brewer's yeast, beer, vinegar [and foods containing vinegar, such as olives, mustard, ketchup, BBQ sauce, and steak sauce] soy sauce, miso, tamari, and fermented products like sauerkraut or kimchee).

It is possible that systematically eliminating these foods even for a short period—letting your body rebalance itself and rest, then re-introducing those foods one at a time, (while carefully monitoring for your reactions)—can lead you to valuable information to include in your personal "body owner's manual" regarding hidden food allergies or sensitivities, and will be well worth the minor inconvenience of having a boring, somewhat bland diet for a few weeks.

In moving toward your best health, you'll find that your body weight will reduce quite naturally (with the addition of exercise, see Chapter 8). As you re-assess your relationship to food and eating, you'll easily make better choices for the benefit of your body, your mind, and the long-range health of both.

Dieting

There is no question that consistent, prolonged stress and the over-production of cortisol play a direct role in weight gain.[2] Dieting is not the answer. Dieting not only brings on stress through feelings of deprivation, reduced energy, and depression, there is also a subliminal stress caused from your body's own quest for the missing nutrients that it needs to function properly. So, dieting causes new stress of its own. *Diets do not work.* They just don't. Here's how they fool you into believing that you're losing weight.

Their trickery is that they are very low in carbohydrates and consequently deplete the healthy glycogen (the storage form of glucose) stores in your muscles and liver used for energy, causing fluid loss from your body. Depletion of your muscle glycogen also leads to muscle atrophy (loss of muscle). This is what you see reflected on your scale, which gets misinterpreted as weight loss when it's actually mostly from dehydration and muscle loss. Once your body gets rehydrated with water, the weight comes right back, except for *the muscle*. Muscle burns fat, so this valuable loss of muscle means that it now becomes even harder for you to actually lose weight. The muscle loss is also indiscriminant. Your heart, being the largest muscle in your body, is not protected in any way from the loss that occurs. This is one of the dangers of so-called "yo-yo dieting"—it can weaken your heart muscle.

Excluding any initial dramatic loss due mostly to losing water weight, a fairly disciplined person can expect to lose between 1 and 2 pounds per week on *any* diet plan or weight loss program according to the American Dietetic Association.[3]

So, what *does* work for effective weight loss?! Work with your doctor, a registered dietician, or nutritionist like myself to develop a personalized eating plan devised for your individual body. The goal is optimizing your health—weight loss will be a natural result.

It's so much more than just balancing calories out and calories in—you must also burn them through optimal forms of movement, which we'll cover in Chapter 6. Whenever possible, try to eat the most nutrient-dense foods that are appealing to you, rather than thinking of it as a diet. You'll develop new and healthier favorites!

What the Heck Is "Nutrient Density"?

To reduce stress, you have to reduce the unconscious stress that happens when you don't properly feed your body. Food is more than medicine—it's information! Its language is all the nutrients, carbohydrates, fats, proteins, and vitamins; dietary minerals, water, and oxygen; carbon, hydrogen, nitrogen, phosphorus, sulfur, calcium, salt, magnesium, and potassium, as well as a host of macronutrients. The food uses are the same DNA letters (G, A, T, and C) that you've come to associate with the genetic code that makes us, "us." That's why you need your body to receive the best quality language—words and phrases that are easy to understand and give your body the kind of information that it can use to keep you healthy.

Nutrient density is that high-quality food information. It's a measure of the amount of nutrients a food contains in comparison with the number of calories it has. The greater the level of nutrients compared to the number of calories, the more nutrient-dense a food is. By choosing the healthiest foods, you'll get all of the essential nutrients, including vitamins, minerals, phytonutrients, essential fatty acids, and fiber, that you need for excellent health and to reduce stress. Here is a peek at the top eight foods.

1. **Spirulina:** This salt water plant has more antioxidants than any other food on Earth and is loaded with protein and minerals. It contains rich vegetable protein (60 to 63 percent, 3 to 4 times higher than fish or beef) and multi-vitamins (vitamin B12 is 3 to 4 times higher than animal liver). It contains a wide range of minerals (including iron, potassium, magnesium sodium, phosphorus, calcium, and so on), a high volume of beta-carotene, which protects cells (5 times more than carrots, 40 times more than spinach), and high volumes of gamma-linolein acid (which can reduce cholesterol and prevent heart disease).

2. **Kale:** Kale is loaded not just with minerals, vitamins, fiber, and amino acids, but also important antioxidants that reduce inflammation. Some researchers believe it can help prevent cancer. Isothiocyanates (ITCs) made from glucosinolates in kale play a principal role in attaining these risk-lowering benefits.

3. **Hemp Seeds:** An amazing natural blend of easily digested proteins, essential fats (Omega 3 and 6), fiber, antioxidants, zinc, iron, carotene, phospholipids, phytosterols, vitamin B1, vitamin B2, vitamin B6, vitamin D, vitamin E, chlorophyll, calcium, magnesium, sulfur, copper, potassium, phosphorus, and enzymes. All of the amino acids essential to optimum health are found in hemp seeds, including the rarely found gamma linolenic acid (GLA). The 17-plus grams of omega fats supplied by hemp seeds provides sufficient, continuous energy throughout your day. This easily digestible seed is versatile, easy to use, and extremely tasty, too. Also, try hemp milk!

4. **Chocolate:** Hold on. Not milk chocolate. We're talking about raw cacao beans or nibs (or really, really dark chocolate). It contains minerals, vitamins, and tons of antioxidants that are great for

your heart and skin, and stimulate your brain to release endorphins that elevate your mood.

5. **Broccoli:** Just a cup of broccoli contains your recommended daily allowance (RDA) of vitamin C; it also fortifies your immune system with a whopping 1,359 mcg of beta-carotene, and small but useful amounts of zinc and selenium (both trace minerals that act as cofactors in numerous immune system defensive actions). Broccoli sprouts are even better!

6. **Spinach:** Loaded with flavonoids that act as antioxidants, spinach protects your body from free radicals (more on this later). Thirteen different flavonoid compounds that act as anti-cancer substances have been discovered by current research. The antioxidants also keep cholesterol from oxidizing. It is also rich in folate, which is good for a healthy cardiovascular system, as well as magnesium (a mineral that assists in lowering high blood pressure).

7. **Chia:** Also high in antioxidants, chia is the richest plant-source of Omega-3, which is important in your heart and cholesterol health. By weight, chia contains more Omega-3 than salmon. It's also great in cleansing your digestive tract and can also help improve elimination.

8. **Berries:** Full of vital vitamins, minerals, and those free-radical avenging antioxidants.

How Are "Phyto" Nutrients Different?

While we can simply come in out of the harsh sun, plants can't move. They can't just flick on air conditioning when it gets too hot or put on sunscreen and sunglasses. So, plants are constantly exposed to damaging radiation, toxins, and pollution. This continual toxic exposure results in the generation of free radicals within their cells. Since plants can't move away from these elements, nature has provided them with a means of protection: they can make a variety of protective compounds called phytonutrients. *Ta-da!*

Phytonutrients are a plant's emergency response team—think of them as the Plant Police, Fire Department, and Coast Guard all rolled into one.

As guardians, phytonutrients protect their plant from free radical attack, from excess ultraviolet radiation, and from predator pests. Phytonutrients do their work with extra *flair*, giving plants sensory characteristics such as scent, color, and flavor.

Almost all plants use sunlight for their energy source. When we think of sunlight, we experience it as a single, bright force, but it's actually made up of many different wavelengths. Plants capture some of these wavelengths to create energy, while other wavelengths can be harmful to the plants.

If a plant was only a single color, with no deviations or shades in that color, then it would only able to receive and protect a single specific wavelength of light. A plant with one color is like a cell phone with a standard antenna, while a plant with many different colors is like a cell phone attached to a satellite tower.

Most plants have a satellite tower's worth of colors—some appear very green to our eyes. But think of it like the primer used beneath a coat of paint; these other colors are there, but they are simply dominated by the primary color you see. Even using ultraviolet light will reveal another amazing dimension of color. Again, each color reflects a different strain of protection.

Antioxidants have been proven to provide protection from potentially damaging free radicals in your body, most of which result from stress of one kind or another (we'll get to that in just a moment). Each plant contains literally thousands of different phytonutrients that can act as antioxidants.

Like plants, we're exposed to ultraviolet radiation or pollution; we also generate reactive, free radicals. Although we can't produce our own phytonutrients, when we eat plants (especially raw), their phytonutrients also protect us against damage from these free radicals.

Free Radicals Are What?

Okay, Biology 101 again. An atom has a central nucleus surrounded by a nice cloud of negatively charged electrons and electrically neutral neutrons. *Remember?* But did you know that the average adult human body contains approximately 6.7×10^{27} atoms and is composed of 60 chemical elements? A whopping 87 percent of human body atoms are either hydrogen or oxygen. *That's a lot of atoms!*

Free radicals are atoms or groups of atoms with an odd (unpaired) number of electrons and can be formed when oxygen interacts with certain molecules. But these free radicals are highly reactive and they can start a chain reaction, like falling dominoes. Not good.

Their leading danger comes from the damage that they can do when they react with important cellular components such as DNA or the cell membrane we talked about earlier. When this happens your cells may function poorly or even die.

In a nutshell, free radicals are reactive molecules that can bind and damage proteins, cell membranes, and DNA.

But, to prevent free radical damage your body has a defense system of *antioxidants*. These are molecules that safely network with free radicals to quickly terminate the destructive chain reaction *before* any crucial molecules are actually damaged.

Although you do have several enzyme systems in your body that scavenge free radicals; the main micronutrient (vitamin) antioxidants are vitamin C, beta-carotene, vitamin E, and selenium.

So the bottom line is: phytonutrients provide plants with protection from the environmental challenges that they are threatened by (like the damage from ultraviolet light). When we eat those plants rich in phytonutrients, they provide us with that same protection as well. This is why covering your plate with colorful fruits and vegetables is so important for your health, well-being, and stress reduction.

What's really significant here is that your body cannot manufacture these micronutrients so they *must be* supplied in your diet through fruits and vegetables (especially raw)!

Why raw? Raw is an easier language for your body to understand. Think of it this way: your body's make-up at its most fundamental is an alphabet soup of information that just happens to be strings of code we call DNA, and plants are too. So when you consume plants in their raw state, your body gets all of that plants' info easily and directly. That information helps your body heal itself and it stabilizes both mental and physical health. *But,* when you cook those veggies (especially when you throw them in a microwave and "nuke" them) the information that they store gets corrupted and much of it is unusable.

Major classes of phytonutrients include:

» **Organosulfurs:** These are the glucobrassicin you'll get from crucifers (asparagus, kale, broccoli, cauliflower, cabbage, Brussels sprouts, turnips, and so on) and the allyl sulfur compounds in garlic.

» **Terpenoids:** This group contains the basic terpenoids like the limonene you find in citrus foods (oranges, mandarins, lemons, tangerines, grape fruits, tangelos, pummelo, kumquats, and limes), menthol (peppermint, spearmint, basil, rosemary, sage, oregano, and catnip), as well as the carotenoids (precursors of Vitamin A), Coenzyme Q10, the tocopherols, tocotrienols, and phytosterols.

» **Flavonoids:** These are the plant pigments that give plants their many colors, like the orange of tangerines, deep blue of blueberries, the green of grapes, or the red of tomatoes. Flavonoids include the quercetin found in onions and anthocyanidins in blueberries.

» **Isoflavonoids and lignans:** Food sources for isoflavone include miso, chickpeas, fava beans, and all members of the legume family. Diadzein is found in the lignans in foods like flaxseed and rye.

» **Organic acids:** One good example would be ferulic acid found in whole grains like corn, buckwheat, oats, black and brown rice, quinoa, amaranth, and whole grain spelt, and coumarins, which you get in foods like parsley, licorice, and citrus fruits.

So here are a few quick ideas to consider as you choose to de-stress, restore, and revitalize that amazing body of yours:

1. Reduce or eliminate your processed food, sugar, and grain carbohydrate intake. Seriously decrease the "white stuff," which means white flour and white sugar, and also includes white rice, cookies, cakes, breads, cereal, granola, and crackers. Yes, this is even true for whole, unprocessed organic grains, because they actually break

down pretty quickly and drive your insulin and leptin levels up, which you don't want.

But don't skip the carbohydrates altogether. Carbohydrates have long been demonized, but your body needs carbs to produce serotonin (the "feel-good" brain chemical that elevates mood, suppresses appetite, and has a calming effect).

In fact, when you cut carbs, you need to replace those calories with healthy fats like avocado, coconut oil, olives, olive oil, and raw nuts (such as almonds or pecans). Also, carbs that you get from most vegetables are quite healthy, though you want to include other carbs in your diet, like black or brown rice in your diet, quinoa, teff, and amaranth.

2. Control your fasting insulin and leptin levels. This is something you'll monitor along with your doctor through simple and relatively inexpensive blood tests.

    Food is fuel; skip a meal and you'll feel tired and cranky. When you go too long without eating, your blood sugar sinks and mood swings follow. Always strive to eat four or five small meals spread throughout your day (instead of the standard two or three larger meals). This will assist your body in maintaining optimal blood sugar levels, which reduces the risk for serious diet-related chronic diseases, including Type-2 diabetes. It will also cut down your cravings for the less healthy choices because your body is so well fed. *There's no room left for junk!* This single action can greatly reduce your everyday stress levels by reducing or eliminating the subliminal stress brought on through low energy levels, sense of deprivation, and your body's urgency for missing nutrients needed to function properly.

3. Eat at least one-third of your food raw. In other words, you've got three things on your plate, one of them should be something raw! (Specifically the family of cruciferous vegetables like broccoli, collards, kale, cabbage, Brussels sprouts, and kohlrabi, unless you have thyroid issues.) Also eat plenty of garlic and onions, which help increase sulfur in the body and aid detoxification. Turmeric, cayenne, ginger, and wasabi are also beneficial.

Remember, when we heat foods we destroy the language in our foods. It gets distorted or muted altogether.

Those with a particularly sensitive digestive system or irritable bowel syndrome, colitis, ulcerative colitis, ileitis, ulcers or Crohn's disease should always use extreme caution with any increase in raw veggies. For some, a significant decrease in stomach flora balance has caused a significant lack of hydrochloric acid, causing difficulty in digesting many things, including raw veggies. In such cases always consult your doctor. It may be necessary to have a week or two of all cooked foods while supplementing with probiotics until the colon is re-lined again, healthy, and able to better digest. There's more on probiotics later.

4. Normalize your ratio of omega-3 to omega-6 fats by taking a high-quality krill oil supplement and reducing (or ideally eliminating) your intake of most processed vegetable oils (canola, corn, peanut, grapeseed, safflower, sunflower, and cottonseed) because these typically raise triglycerides, a fatty substance in the blood, and lowers HDL, increasing the risk of cardiovascular disease. Research suggests that low omega-3 levels are associated with depression, pessimism, and impulsivity—all things that add to stress.

Extra-virgin olive oil is a better monounsaturated fat and works great as a salad dressing. However, it is *not* the best oil to cook with. This is simply because of its chemical structure, which makes it susceptible to oxidative damage when heated.

Coconut oil is by far your best choice for cooking. It is unique in its high concentration of medium chain fatty acids (MCFA's) at 62 percent. Also, because it helps to stimulate your metabolism, you may burn more calories each day, helping to *accelerate weight loss* (and helps your energy levels too). Coconut oil has often been compared to carbohydrates in its ability to be "burned" for energy. However, since insulin is not involved in the process of digesting the MCFA's in coconut oil, you won't get those carb-related spikes in your blood sugar level, which is really good news for anyone concerned about maintaining normal blood sugar levels.

5. Avoid frying, grilling, or charbroiling your food. AGE, HCA, and PAH are all carcinogens formed when meat is cooked at high temperatures. Also, the higher the temperature at which the food is cooked, the longer it stays in your gut and the more difficult it becomes to digest.

    Simply put, overcooking makes it more difficult for its nutrients to be absorbed and function at the cellular level needed to produce energy. When food cannot function in your cells, the cells can become deficient or possibly toxic, which then leads to deficiency and toxicity within your body as a whole. This not only makes your body less able to function optimally, but becomes its own source of stress. Boil, sauté, poach, or steam your foods instead.

6. Ideally, you should move your bowels daily. The wonderful ratio of fruits and vegetables you're eating should make this quite simple. This should happen effortlessly—don't force it. Any disruption of your digestive cycle, such as constipation, allows harmful bacteria to hang around longer, which also allows them to proliferate (causing all manner of issues).

Are Nutritional Supplements Really Necessary?

Once we pass the age of 25 or so, our bodies simply do not have the capacity to absorb nutrients from our foods in the necessary amounts for good health—and the foods we have access to in our stores are woefully lacking in beneficial nutrient levels by the time they reach our kitchen.

There are those who espouse the belief that vitamins are a complete waste of money. They're right, if:

»   That's true *if*, and only *if*, you eat a consistent diet of non-genetically modified, fresh, whole, organic, locally farmed food that is grown in pristine, non-toxic, mineral and nutrient-rich soils; given clean water; and not stored for months before eaten.

»   It's also true only *if* you live and work outside in the "Goldilocks zone" between zero degrees to around 35 degrees north of the

Earth's equator, which is drenched in sunshine; drink only pure, unpolluted water; breath only fresh clean air; sleep soundly for a full nine hours nightly; exercise your body every day; are free from chronic stressors and contact with any environmental toxins; are in a loving, fulfilling, supportive relationship; involved in enlivening, educational, and inspiring activities; and have a deep connected inner spiritual relationship.

If that sounds like your lifestyle, then you don't need vitamins! The problem is that hardly *any* of us live this way. In fact, more than 92 percent of Americans are deficient in at least one vitamin or mineral—and that's in the minimum amounts needed to prevent disease caused by deficiencies! Now factor in the poor intestinal absorption rate (which naturally declines as we advance in age), and you've got older folks barely getting any nutrients at all.

So give serious consideration to supplementation, which will assist your body in functioning optimally without the stress of it having to stretch its very limited resources in trying to stay energetic, vibrant, and *healthy*!

Talking With Your Doctor

A good quality multi-vitamin is a place to start. Consider a calcium (as citrate) supplement, which has an equal ratio of magnesium (this balance is necessary for your body to absorb it; also, it is best taken with citrus). Vitamin C supplementation is also vital to maintaining optimal health along with vitamin E, which is a powerful antioxidant and supports respiratory and heart health. Omega 3 (as krill oil) supports both cardiovascular and joint health. Chlorella reportedly helps detoxify your body and rids the body of toxins present in your food, as well as in the environment. Coenzyme Q10 (Ubiquinol) is an antioxidant, which also increases cell energy production, as well as free radical elimination. Also consider grape seed extract, which reportedly prevents formation of plaque in arteries, increases circulation, and improves mental alertness. Further, you'll want to consider normalizing your Vitamin D3 levels.

Other supplements to look into would be alpha lipoic acid, N-acetyl cysteine, L-arginine, and L-carnitine. You can learn more about these in the Appendix. Please remember, any supplementation should be discussed with and monitored by your physician.

Digestive Enzymes: Why You Need Them

All of the metabolic functions in your body are directed by enzymes. This means simply that your stamina, your energy level, your ability to utilize vitamins and minerals, your immune system, and your elimination of waste are all run by enzymes.

Digestive enzymes in particular are produced both internally (mainly in your pancreas and other endocrine glands) and are present in the wonderful raw veggies that you eat. They allow the nutrients from your food to be easily absorbed into the bloodstream and used for all of your body functions.

Since most of us do not bother (or have time) to really *chew our food*, the pre-digestion phase of our whole digestion process is pretty lame. This leaves our pancreas and the other organs of the endocrine system under incredible strain in order to draw reserves from your entire body to produce massive amounts of the proper digestive enzymes needed.

According to Dr. Edward Howell, author of *Enzyme Nutrition*, when we're born, we have a certain limited potential for naturally manufacturing them; let's call it an enzyme "reserve." Studies have shown that every 10 years, your body's production of enzymes decreases by 13 percent.[4] So let's add that up. By age 40, your enzyme production could be 25 percent lower than it was when you were a kid, and by the time you're 70, well, you could be producing only one-third of the digestive enzymes you actually need. It would seem that nature intended for us to continually replenish our reserve through good nutrition and eating habits. Unfortunately, it didn't foresee our modern eating habits, farming techniques, and oh, yes, *STRESS*!

Research has shown definitively that your intestines responds negatively to stress.[5] Your gut is extremely vulnerable to stress-induced changes in your secretion of necessary gastric fluids, digestion responsiveness, and also the permeability and barrier function allowing you to get nutrients through and keep toxins out (called "leaky gut"). There has even been evidence to suggest that your gut microbiota may respond directly to stress-related host signals. That's right! Even the microscopic bacteria in your intestines are listening and responding to your stress as it ebbs and flows.

Dr. Candace Pert wrote an amazing book called *The Molecules of Emotion* in which she details her research about neurotransmitters (brain-produced signaling molecules) found surrounding your entire intestinal tract, which were once believed to only exist in our brains.[6]

Furthermore, neurotransmitter receptors, which can bind and respond to these signaling molecules, are also located all along your intestinal tract. Therefore, it is known that brain signaling molecules can easily affect your intestinal tract. Foods with a calming effect include herbal teas, such as chamomile. Alcohol, caffeine, and refined carbohydrates, such as table sugar, should be avoided. Eating meals at regular times and in a *relaxed environment* can also help decrease *STRESS*.

On average, food travels through your stomach anywhere between 30 minutes to two hours, continues through the small intestine during the next two to six hours, and spends six to 72 hours in your large intestine before final removal by defecation. The less digestion that takes place before food reaches your small intestine, the greater the strain placed on your endocrine system. Oh, and don't forget what stress in your life has already done to reduce the efficiency of your digestion.

Pancreatic cancer is now number 4 on the list in the United States, accounting for more than 29,000 deaths each year.[7] For reasons unexplained, there has been a three-fold increase in pancreatic cancer in the last 40 years. This could contribute to our diabetes epidemic.[8]

Low stomach acid (hypochlorhydria) is common, especially in older people, because, as we age, we make less stomach acid. Research suggests that as many as 30 percent of the people over 60 years old have hypochlorhydria.[9]

There are so many factors that can and do inhibit your adequate stomach acid production including *Helicobacter pylori* (*H. pylori*), pathogenic bacteria, and frequent use of antacids. Hypochlorhydria is also associated with many diseases, such as rheumatoid arthritis, osteoporosis, asthma, celiac sprue, hepatitis, and diabetes mellitus. Signs of hypochlorhydria include bloating, indigestion, excessive belching, multiple food allergies, undigested food in the stool, and cracked or peeling fingernails. In addition to hydrochloric acid, some peoples' production of pancreatic enzymes and bicarbonate are also compromised.

So, by simply using digestive enzymes with your meals, you'll use up far less of your body's natural limited reserve and help with the all-important digestion process. When foods are not well-digested, digestion slows. Not good. This results in a build-up of waste in your colon. The fecal matter begins to decay, producing bacteria and toxins. The toxins will ultimately seep through your bowel wall, where blood capillaries transport and distribute them throughout the body. This can result in a multitude of health problems, such as: constipation, stomach bloat, poor digestion, gas, fatigue, weight gain, headaches, and more.

Using digestive enzymes with your meals will ensure that your foods are more completely digested. Oh, and *CHEW*!

You'll want to speak with your doctor, but consider a vegetarian-based digestive enzyme supplement that contains a variety of proteases, including:

- » Papain aids in the digestion of protein. Made from papaya, it's so effective in digesting proteins that it's often used as a meat tenderizer.
- » Amylase for digestion of starches and carbohydrates.
- » Lipase to digest fats.
- » Cellulase, which is invaluable in breaking down fiber cellulose into smaller units.
- » Lactase, which works in the digestion of dairy products.
- » Bromelain, which comes from pineapple stalks, is a miracle enzyme. It digests protein, and it burns 900 times its weight in fat, and it's amazingly beneficial for the body as a whole once it gets into your bloodstream, particularly in terms of reducing inflammation and swelling in joints.

For consistent issues with indigestion, another option is to take a betaine hydrochloric supplement, which is available in health food stores without a prescription. After discussing this option with your doctor, they'll suggest that you initially take enough to get the slightest burning sensation and then decrease by one capsule. This will help your body to better digest your food, and will also help kill *helicobacter pylori* and normalize your symptoms. This is not a long-term supplement, but you'll also be simultaneously working toward balancing your stomach pH and using probiotics. *Did I mention chewing?!*

Why Probiotics Rock!

Alright, so you know what an antibiotic is. You've got that one down. Anytime you have an infection the doctor writes a "script" for an antibiotic to kill off the nasty bacteria. Your body actually contains approximately 100 trillion bacteria—that's more than 10 *times* the number of cells you have. You have about three pounds worth of bacteria sitting right there in your colon. So the next time you step on the scale to weigh yourself, be sure to deduct your passengers!

Probiotics are a type of "good" bacteria. The ideal ratio between the bacteria in your body is 85 percent "good" to 15 percent "bad." Signs and symptoms that you may need to address your intestinal balance include nausea, gas and bloating, constipation or diarrhea, headaches, fatigue, sugar cravings, and cravings for refined carb foods (chips, fries, breads, and so on).

Did you know that 80 percent of your whole immune system is located right there in your gut? Let's take a guess at what's in your colon to make sure everything goes right. *Yep!* Probiotics are in there managing the proper development and function of your immune system as well as protection against over-growth of other microorganisms that could cause disease.

But wait, there's more! Probiotics naturally create *antibiotics* made to precisely act on specific invaders (pathogens). Whenever the invader becomes resistant to that antibiotic, the probiotic will then produce a new, even more effective antibiotic. This is in total contrast to oral prescribed antibiotics, which can become resistant to pathogens through time and be ineffective, allowing invaders to take hold in your body.

That's not all, folks! These microorganisms help with digestion of food and absorption of nutrients.

Kinda gives you a little more respect for your tiny buggers, doesn't it? The beneficial microorganisms that normally inhabit your colon are pretty well-established shortly after birth and will remain reasonably stable throughout your life. However, on a daily basis that vital and delicate balance of bacteria in your intestines can be thrown off-kilter through external challenges. Ensuring that you're getting a regular supply of good bacteria in your digestive system to keep it balanced is crucial to your health.

What is it that makes your gut bacteria lose balance?

» Antibiotics, whether therapeutic or consumed indirectly through our food supply, are the single largest offender in encouraging overgrowth of harmful pathogens in your gastrointestinal tract (a condition called dysbiosis) that may be the source of many autoimmune disorders and certain cancers. The issue here is that antibiotics exterminate both bad and friendly bacteria indiscriminately. This allows dangerous strains of harmful microorganisms to thrive.

» Heartburn meds can be harmful to your gut flora, such as Alka-Seltzer, Alka-2, Surpass Gum, Titralac, Tums, Alternagel, Amphojel, Gaviscon, Gelusil, Maalox, Mylanta, Rolaids, Pepto-Bismol, Axid AR, Pepcid AC, Tagamet HB, Zantac 75, Tolmetin (Tolectin), Nexium, Prilosec, Protonix, Aciphex, and Prevacid.

» Chemotherapy and radiation are equally devastating to bacterial flora.

» Non-steroidal anti-inflammatory drugs (NSAIDS) like Celebrex, Advil, Aleve, Motrin, Midol, and Aspirin are all damaging to healthy balanced intestinal flora.

» Antibacterial soap.

» Cigarettes.

» Alcohol.

» Stress.

» Chlorine in your everyday drinking water not only kills the unwelcome bacteria, it's equally devastating to healthy colonies of beneficial bacteria living in your intestines.

» Aging. Even colonies of beneficial bacteria will eventually lose their vitality.

» Fertilizers, pesticides, and other agricultural chemicals used on our food crops.

» Virtually all non-organic meat, poultry, and dairy that you eat are unfortunately laden with antibiotics.

» High-protein diets. Protein takes longer to break down in your body. This supports the growth of detrimental, putrefying bacteria.

» Constipation allows harmful bacteria to linger longer, allowing them to proliferate.

You can easily see now why supplementation with a good probiotic is mandatory to elevate your standard of health. In order to have true health or recovery from disease, you must have healthy colonies of more than 100 trillion beneficial microorganisms happily thriving in your intestinal tract. It honestly is that simple. They support digestion, nutrient absorption, and the production of significant amounts of vitamins and enzymes, while working to crowd out harmful bacteria by denying them space to flourish.

So what are the benefits of strengthening and optimizing your digestive track?

» Preservation of an ideal ratio of good to bad bacteria.

» Benefits in metabolism.

» Break-down of toxins.

» Protection against food poisoning.

» Bolsters normal inflammatory response.

» Creation of lactic acid for support of digestive processes and colonic pH balance.

» Lowered cholesterol (through support of protein and carbohydrate digestion).

» Potential cancer inhibition.

» Maintenance of appropriate serum lipid and blood pressure levels.
» Protection against lactose and casein intolerance.
» Protection from candida overgrowth and vaginal yeast infections.
» Correction and prevention of irritable bowel syndrome (IBS), colitis, constipation, diarrhea, ileitis, stomach ulcers, and a whole range of other digestive tract dysfunctions, as well as maintaining appropriate bowel transit time.
» Enhancement in the health and appearance of the skin.
» Improvement of absorption and the internal generation of vitamin K and B vitamins.

You will want to increase your probiotic (good bacteria) intake with a high-quality probiotic supplement or by eating certain cultured and fermented foods, such as organic Kefir, Natto, Miso, Kimchi, Sauerkraut, or organic Greek Yogurt.

What to Look for in a Probiotic Supplement

It's more than a little daunting to see the hundreds of probiotic supplement products on the market today. They're everywhere—from powders and capsules, to foods, such as yogurt, dairy drinks, infant formulas, cheese, and some snack bars. Of course, all of these probiotic supplements were not created equal. Probiotic supplements can vary widely in colony forming units (CFU) of bacteria used in promoting a healthier digestive tract. Only clinically proven products should truly be called probiotic. A good probiotics manufacturer will label their probiotic product with the following information for you:

1. Contents should show the genus, species, and strain of probiotic.
2. Make sure the formula you choose includes the all-important supernatant. (This simply refers to the medium the culture was grown in. The supernatant itself contains a multitude of beneficial byproducts of the growth process, including vitamins, enzymes, antioxidants, and immune stimulators.)
3. Listed on the product should be the minimum numbers of viable bacteria at the *end* of shelf life. The die-off rate for probiotics is

ridiculously high. Pick up any probiotic formula and check out the label. You'll see wording like "Contains 13 billion live organisms per capsule at time of manufacture." And that's the problem: "at time of manufacture."

4. Quality probiotic product will have guaranteed levels of live bacteria at the point of consumption rather than at the point of manufacture.

5. Look for a product that has a "use by" or expiration date stated clearly on the package.

6. Advice for proper storage conditions.

7. Corporate contact details for consumer information.

8. Refrigeration information. During shipment and storage, products have often been exposed to warm temperatures that will kill off some (or even all) of the bacteria.

9. Be certain to choose a product that has an enteric coating, which is a barrier applied to oral medication that controls the location in the digestive system where it is absorbed. "Enteric" refers to the small intestine, therefore enteric coatings prevent release of medication before it reaches the small intestine.

There are many beneficial bacteria that you may find contained within a good probiotic, but two are dominant. Look for a formula based on these elements:

» *L. acidophilus* lives primarily in your small intestine and produces a number of potent antimicrobial compounds (including acidolin, acidolphilin, lactocidin, and bacteriocin). These compounds can limit growth and toxin-producing abilities of a minimum of 23 known disease-causing pathogens (including campylobacter, listeria, and staphylococci), as well as decrease tumor growth and effectively neutralize or obstruct carcinogenic substances.

Another significant note: *L. acidophilus* is the primary helpful bacteria in the vaginal tract. When the acidophilus balance is disrupted, this allows culprits such as gardnerella vaginalis, E. coli, or chlamydia to proliferate.

» **Bifidobacteria** level stability in the large intestine. Many researchers believe this essentially marks the beginnings of chronic degenerative disease. Bifidobacteria benefit your body in many ways. They actually consume old fecal matter, have the capability to remove cancer-forming elements (or the enzymes that lead to their formation), and have been found to protect against the formation of liver, colon, and mammary gland tumors.

Glutamine

Glutamine is simply the most abundant amino acid found in your body and is primarily located in the lining of your small intestine, which is right where the nutrients are absorbed.

Glutamine is the major component in making essential neurotransmitters. Research has confirmed real improvements in memory retention, cognitive ability, and problem-solving when glutamine was supplemented in the diet. Glutamine assists your body in maintaining constant blood sugar levels. This is an absolute necessity for optimal brain function because in addition to oxygen, that brain of yours uses glucose (blood sugar) as its primary source of fuel.

Glutamine contributes a significant role in maintaining healthy muscle metabolism during stress, illness, and exercise. It enables removal of toxic ammonia from your liver. (Rather than being converted into harmful ammonia, the additional nitrogen in the liver attaches itself to glutamic acid to form glutamine). And glutamine is also an important precursor to the antioxidant glutathione, which participates in glycogen synthesis (the storage form of carbohydrate), and provides nitrogen compounds for the production of nucleotides (used to make DNA and RNA).

This all sounds great, right? Well, here's the thing. Stressful conditions, including surgery, fasting, or improper eating habits consistently reduce your intramuscular glutamine levels. Also, your emotional stress discharges hormones (glucocorticoids, epinephrine, glucagon), which will cause a significant reduction in intramuscular glutamine by stimulating both muscle glutamine synthesis and permitting the escape of this amino acid from skeletal muscle. *Not good.*

For one thing, your gastrointestinal tract simply cannot function without glutamine. It encourages your healthy digestion by assisting in the delicate pH balance of acid/alkaline levels in your body. Glutamine from foods (such as organic chicken, fish, beans, parsley, cabbage, and spinach—raw veggies having better quantities than cooked) can be absorbed directly into the cells of your small intestine and may be a big help for people who have trouble absorbing nutrients due to compromised digestion. Glutamine is a primary treatment for ulcers and disorders of the small and large intestine such as colitis or irritable bowel syndrome (IBS) characterized by constipation, diarrhea, or both. It is believed by some health professionals that glutamine supplements may benefit people with intestinal problems such as ileitis, ulcers, and Crohn's disease.

Do you see the wide variety of negative effects stress—which most of us experience on a daily basis to some degree—can have on large areas of your health?

Your moods, attitudes, and reactions to the environment around you will directly affect not only your digestion, but your body's ability to metabolize the food that you've eaten. This vital link between your nervous system and your digestive system has been fully documented in recent years. A constant exchange of chemicals and electrical messages between the two systems happens instantaneously. Many scientists now refer to them as one entity: the "brain-gut axis." Yep, what affects your stomach will directly affect your brain and vice versa.

Your brain and digestive system are connected. What you feel and think has direct effects, influencing the release of proteins that interact with your nervous system (neuropeptides), which in turn will affect your intestinal motility, secretion, blood flow, and inflammation. Stress influences your inflammatory pathways, which lead to dysregulation that can cause emotional conditions and even more stress. This becomes a vicious cycle.

Serotonin has been labeled "the feel-good" hormone. Guess what? About 95 percent of your body's serotonin is located in your gut, where it acts as a neurotransmitter and a signaling mechanism. In fact, nearly every chemical that controls your brain is also located in your stomach region, including hormones and neurotransmitters such as serotonin, dopamine, glutamate, GABA, and Norepinephrine. Your serotonin receptors are involved in a variety of vital processes, including mood, memory, sleep, learning, cognition, thermo-regulation, appetite, anxiety, depression, bowel movements, and nausea. This gives new meaning to the phrase "gut feeling."

Your serotonin levels are directly affected by your diet. An increase in the ratio of tryptophan to phenylalanine and leucine will increase serotonin levels. Fruits that have a good ratio of these include bananas, dates, and papayas. Foods with a lower ratio will inhibit your production of serotonin. These include rye and whole wheat bread. *Sorry!*

Your muscles use many of the amino acids with the exception of tryptophan, which is important because this allows more muscular individuals to produce more serotonin. It gives you another reason to both eat right and to exercise. *Right!?*

Can't I Just Use Antacids to Improve My Digestion?

Nope! We tend to take these drugs lightly. So often when we are under stress, stomach acid just seems to build and we reach for what we believe will be a quick fix. Antacids are so commonplace that we use them for all manner of stomach discomfort—acid indigestion, upset stomach, sour stomach, and heartburn. Additional components of some formulations include dimethicone to reduce gas pains (flatulence) and alginic acid, which, in combination with antacids, may help manage gastro-esophageal reflux disease (GERD). Some people pop them like candy and even use them as breath fresheners, but they are *real* medications with *real* consequences. Used only occasionally, they do no real harm, but if you're living on them, they will have serious side effects that will bring you even more stress.

In the end, they just mask your symptoms of indigestion, heartburn, or acid reflux, and do absolutely nothing to repair your real underlying problem. In fact, they actually make your problem worse in the long run. How? Antacids work on the principle that alkalis cancel out acids. Simple translation: they are stomach acid neutralizers (but even at that they are only effective until the alkalizing ingredients in them are used up in just a few hours), but their effects can go much deeper.

Here's the problem: *Any* time the acid level in your stomach is reduced, you run the risk of not digesting your food properly (causing more digestive problems) and the risk of nutrients from your food not being absorbed by the body.

To make matters even worse, the natural acid levels in your stomach are also there to kill off bacteria, viruses, and germs that you ingest every single day. This means low levels of stomach acid can lead to increased infections. *How?*

Biology 101: A healthy pH environment (that is, acid to alkaline balance) in your stomach will digest meats and other proteins and break them down for you into their amino acid components so that your body can absorb these wonderful tissue-building particles that assist in the manufacture and release of vitamins and minerals from the foods you eat. This food is then released into the first part of the small intestine (called the duodenum) through the pyloric valve, where it is combined with more alkaline digestive enzymes from your pancreas and gallbladder, creating a higher pH. This is all great stuff.

But (you knew it was coming) if your stomach pH gets higher than 3.0, it secretes more acid in an effort to return your pH below 3.0. So when heartburn or acid reflux medication that interferes with your natural stomach acid by raising the pH above 3.0, your stomach is no longer functioning like a stomach. It then creates chemical combinations that are not usable by your body, which in turn creates even more problems for the rest of your digestive track, because it has to work that much harder when the food particles are not broken down. Another domino effect takes place.

When that happens, fermentation occurs, which creates more gas and more bloating, *and* some of these indigested food particles can cross the membranes of the intestine (called "leaky gut"), ultimately causing your body to actually become allergic to many foods that you would normally be able to digest with a healthy stomach pH. When you suppress your natural stomach acids, you will not only increase your risk of stomach atrophy, but also virtually every other chronic degenerative disease.

As we discussed earlier, 80 percent of your immune system is located right there in your gut. Reducing the acid in your stomach diminishes your primary defense mechanism for food-borne infections, which will increase your risk of food poisoning and also your risk of infection with *clostridium difficile*, (a harmful intestinal bacterium that is particularly common among the elderly).

Reduced stomach acid leads to IBS, gluten allergies, Crohn's, and a host of other allergy symptoms. Did you just throw your antacids out? Also, some antacids not only cause stomach cramping, but also contain ingredients that can cause constipation, such as aluminum, or diarrhea, such as magnesium.

Can you stand just a little more bad news on antacids? The FDA actually issued a report cautioning against the prolonged use of a class of acid-stopping drugs called proton-pump inhibitors (PPIs). This includes prescription brands such as Nexium and Prilosec (an older generic treatment that is also available over the counter at lower dosage strength). Other proton-pump inhibitors used to treat heartburn, known formally as gastroesophageal reflux disease (GERD), include generically available Protonix, Aciphex, and Prevacid.

According to Mitchell Katz, director of the San Francisco Department of Public Health, PPI's were never intended for people with heartburn, and according to Katz, "about 60 to 70 percent of people taking these drugs have mild heartburn and shouldn't be on them."[10]

The FDA report cautions against high doses or prolonged use of PPI's, because they've been shown to increase the risk of:

» Bone loss.
» Bone fractures.
» Infection.
» Pneumonia.
» Dementia.

The risk of a bone fracture has been estimated to be more than 40 percent higher in patients who use these drugs long-term, which again applies to many seniors.

All acid-stopping drugs (not just PPIs) inhibit your stomach's vital nutrient absorption, promote bacterial overgrowth, reduce resistance to infection, and increase your risk of cancer and other serious diseases. You want to limit their usage or support, and improve your digestion through a balanced diet.

What to Eat? (Glad You Asked!)

Stress requires that you feed your body well to maintain your health. It's simple: good, fresh, organic, locally grown food and clean water. What's that? You don't live on a farm?! Try to find a farmer's market in your area to support, and nag the produce manager at your local store about getting more organics in stock. You may have to shop outside of your neighborhood (travel time and expense then add to your food budget). Eating better does require planning and preparation, and it is well worth the extra effort to feel and see the health benefits. This should not add to your stress—make gradual changes and you'll still see results.

Fact: Eating at least one-third of your diet as raw food is good. An even better choice is to eat a diet based on 80 percent fresh, organic vegetables, seeds, raw nuts, and a little organic fruit, because this helps to put your body into an alkaline environment (meaning it's very balanced and *very* happy). This gets back to the earlier point about the best language from foods to communicate with your body. Your organic vegetables provide you with live enzymes and phytonutrients that are easily absorbed by your body and reach down to the cellular level to nourish and enhance growth of healthy, new cells and keep your body's stress level down.

About 20 percent of your diet can be from cooked food (including beans and legumes, whole grain breads, pastas, and black or brown rice).

Raw is an important factor in your vegetable choice, because it provides essential dietary fiber to assist in proper digestion and good bowel habits. You probably chuckled at this when I mentioned it earlier, but it will make a huge difference in your health.

Enzymes and phytonutrients are destroyed at temperatures of 104 degrees F (40 degrees C), so cooked vegetables (which do provide good dietary fiber) still don't contain as much of the valuable nutrients and none of the enzymes that your body needs. The same, by the way, applies to frozen vegetables. Now just imagine how this information applies to those yummy frozen meals that you nuke in your microwave! Yep! The cardboard box it came in is almost equal in nutritional value.

Studies reveal that when you eat a majority of cooked foods, you are consuming acidic toxins faster than your body can eliminate them, which disrupts your body's delicate pH acid/alkaline balance, becoming a major contributor to not only disease, but also excess weight gain.[11] Heating food above 118 degrees F (47.78 degrees C) causes chemical changes that create acidic toxins, including the free-radicals, carcinogens, and mutagens associated with diseases such as arthritis, diabetes, heart disease, and cancer.

What to Avoid

The first food to avoid is sugar. According to breast cancer expert, author, and board certified surgeon Dr. Christine Horner, "To me, sugar has no redeeming value at all, because they found that the more we consume it, the more we're fuelling every single chronic disease." She continued, "In fact, there was a study done about a year ago (2011) and the conclusion was that sugar is a universal mechanism for chronic disease. It kicks up inflammation. It kicks up oxygen free radicals. Those are the two main processes we see that underlie any single chronic disorder, including cancers. It fuels the growth of breast cancers, because glucose is cancer's favorite food. The more you consume, the faster it grows."[12] *Enough said? Could the message be any clearer?*

By getting rid of sugar (including fructose and high-fructose corn syrup) it cuts off an important food supply to tissue inflammation and to cancer cells. Reduce the amount of overt sugar you get through consuming fruit and fruit juices, and of course all those sugary treats. Sugar substitutes such as NutraSweet, Equal, Spoonful, and so on are made with aspartame, which is extremely harmful. A better natural substitute would be monk fruit extract, stevia, manuka honey, or molasses, but still, *only in very small amounts*.

Also keep an eye on the amount of hidden sugar you intake through foods such as potatoes, tomatoes, squash, and carrots.

The second item is milk. It has been estimated that 75 percent of the world's population is genetically lactose intolerant and do not produce the enzyme necessary to properly digest milk, as well as other dairy products. Research shows that higher intakes of dairy products may increase a man's risk of prostate cancer by anywhere from 30 to 50 percent.

Plus, dairy consumption increases the body's level of insulin-like growth factor-1 (IGF-1)—a known cancer promoter. There's absolutely no evidence that dairy is good for your bones or prevents osteoporosis—in fact, the animal protein that it contains may help *cause* bone loss! Also, according to the Harvard Nurses' Health Study, which investigated the milk-drinking habits of 72,000 women for 12 years, dairy may increase risk of fractures by 50 percent.[13]

By reducing milk and substituting with hemp milk or unsweetened almond milk, cancer cells are being starved. Hemp milk is rich in omega 3 fatty acids, which are great for your heart and your brain. Almond milk is rich in calcium, magnesium, potassium, manganese, copper, vitamin E, and selenium. Both are good for drinking, as well as a good dairy substitute in cooking.

The third food to avoid is unfermented soy products such as tofu, soy milk, soy ice cream, soy cheese, soy nut butters, soy flour, textured soy protein (TSP), texturized vegetable protein (TVP), atsuage, aburage, soybean oil, and yuba. Because of our processing methods, most of today's soy foods are chockfull of toxins, anti-nutrients, and disruptive plant estrogens that have been linked to health issues like malnutrition, digestive problems, reproductive disorders, thyroid dysfunction, cognitive decline, immune system breakdowns, heart disease, and cancer.

Non-fermented soy products contain phytic acid, which binds with certain important nutrients, such as iron, inhibiting their absorption. Expanding on the earlier point, the isoflavones contained in soy are similar to estrogen in chemical structure and can interfere with a woman's natural estrogen production. This not only poses a threat to women, children, and thyroid health in general, but some feel that soy's phytoestrogens may attenuate testosterone levels in boys. Most doctors already advise pregnant women against consuming too much soy.

However, after a long fermentation process, the phytic acid and anti-nutrient levels of soybeans are diminished and their beneficial properties—such as the creation of natural probiotics—become available to your digestive system. This makes fermented soy products, such as brewed soy sauce, tempeh, miso, and tamari, safe and even beneficial to consume.

Red meat is the fourth product on the list. A meat-based diet is acidic. Meat also harbors livestock antibiotics, growth hormones, and parasites, all of which are harmful, especially to people under stress, which lowers immune function. Cancer cells thrive in an acidic environment. Pork is essentially good protein from a biochemical perspective, but there is *more* than enough scientific evidence to justify the reservations or absolute prohibitions across many cultures against eating it. When you cook pork, even for long periods, it is still not enough to kill many of the retroviruses and other parasites that many of them store.

All meat protein is difficult to digest and therefore requires an increase of digestive enzymes. Including digestive enzyme supplements in the diet of habitual red meat eaters is essential.

That said, eliminating animal foods from your diet completely will lead to a low dietary intake of sulfur amino acids and protein, which can increase your risk of heart disease. It may also lead to a serious deficiency in vitamin B12.

According to Sally Fallon, author of *Eat Fat, Lose Fat*, "Not only is it difficult to obtain adequate protein on a diet devoid of animal products, but such a diet often leads to deficiencies in many important minerals as well. This is because a largely vegetarian diet lacks the fat-soluble catalysts needed for mineral absorption."[14]

When you look at a typical vegan diet, you'll notice immediately that it's high in grains. An assumption to draw from this would be that it should contribute to increased levels of iron and phosphorus, but hair sample analysis proves that these minerals aren't absorbed on a cellular level. The excess iron in the vegetarian digestive tract unfortunately works against them by preventing the absorption of selenium and zinc. There is a particular form of iron called "heme," which is found only in the muscle cells and red blood cells of animal protein. It is crucial, abundant, and necessary for energy metabolism at the cellular level, but is absent from vegetarian diets. The high phytic acid intake in vegetarian diets also increases a likelihood of deficiencies in chromium, vanadium, and lithium.

It is best to eat cold-water fish (wild salmon, halibut, sardines, cod, and black cod, or sable) and a little turkey, ostrich, or chicken (free range and organic), rather than beef, bison, or pork. Protein from animal sources need not be eaten every day! Once or twice a week is sufficient.

Our society, along with portion sizes, also has a misconception about meal composition. A person's required protein intake varies. It depends on sex, height, weight, and exercise levels. Normal protein intake ranges from 20 to 50 grams each meal. Women are notoriously deficient in protein consumption. A 45-year-old woman needs 2 to 3 ounces of protein per meal, depending upon activity level. That's equivalent to half of a small chicken breast and a half cup of cooked black beans.

High-protein diets, such as the Atkins diet, may accelerate kidney disease in people at risk. Because proteins must be broken down into amino acids in the body, and waste products excreted, too much protein puts a strain on the body's ability to get rid of waste products, especially in those who already have a kidney problem. Calcium loss, which leads to osteoporosis, also occurs with high levels of protein intake.

The fifth food item to avoid is wheat products. The wheat-based products we currently eat are not made with the heirloom wheat that our grandparents ate. Developed by Nobel laureate Norman Borlaug, the dwarf wheat now farmed around the world contains 28, or twice as many chromosomes, and produces a hefty assortment of gluten proteins, including those most likely to cause celiac disease. It contains a starch called amylopectin A, which actually causes weight gain and a form of super gluten that is highly inflammatory in the body.

It's best to avoid products with gluten, such as wheat, rye, barley, spelt, triticale, and kamut. Here's why. Gluten itself is just a protein, but it's hard to digest and therefore can irritate not only your digestive tract but your other organs as well. It can often pass through your digestive tract undigested. You can experience symptoms such as gas, abdominal distention, abdominal pain, nausea, flatulence, muscle fatigue, pain, or even depression. You may also have gluten sensitivity, but show no overt symptoms whatsoever.

Research shows that as many as 90 million Americans may be negatively affected by gluten and as many as 10 million may be grappling with an illness that stems from gluten sensitivity. So, minimize or completely eliminate wheat if your diet all together. In addition to very obvious foods such as bread, pasta, flour, cereal, crackers, biscuits, rolls, buns, donuts, cakes, and cookies, gluten can be found as a sub-ingredient in salad dressings, BBQ sauce, pickled products, sauces, soy sauce, sausage, soups, stocks, broth, spice and herb blends, hydrolyzed vegetable protein (HVP) textured soy protein (TSP), texturized vegetable protein (TVP), and monosodium glutamate (MSG).

Fluoride is the sixth item to avoid. The practice of water fluoridation has been rejected or banned in several countries, including China, Austria, Belgium, Finland, Germany, Denmark, Norway, Sweden, the Netherlands, Hungary, and Japan. *And guess what?* Research proves that they've experienced the exact same decline in dental decay as the United States.

Unfortunately, the United States' water fluoridation programs do not use chemicals that are of the pharmaceutical grade used in the research, which in 1945 concluded that fluoride reduced tooth decay. Instead, they are using industrial grade by-products from the wet scrubbing systems of the superphosphate fertilizer industry. These chemicals (90 percent of which are hexafluorosilicic acid, sodium fluorosilicate, and fluorosilicic acid), are classified hazardous wastes contaminated with various impurities. Testing done recently by the National Sanitation Foundation suggests that the levels of arsenic in these chemicals are pretty high (up to 1.6 ppb after dilution into public water) and of potential concern.

We also have to consider the effects from chronic fluoride exposure over a long period of time, effects that might be delayed or occur late in life. Research now shows that fluoride accumulates in the brain and exposure alters mental behavior in a manner consistent with a neurotoxic agent. In other words, it is no coincidence that fluoride is one of the basic ingredients in both Prozac (fluoxetene hydrochloride) and Sarin nerve gas (isopropyl-methyl-phosphoryl fluoride). A 2001 study by Jennifer Luke showed that fluoride accumulates in the human pineal gland at very high levels. In her research, Luke demonstrated that fluoride reduces melatonin production and leads to an earlier onset of puberty.

Fluoride exposure also disrupts the synthesis of collagen. Why is that important? Collagen makes up about 25 to 35 percent of your whole-body protein count. Collagen is a vital part of your connective tissue that in the skin assists with firmness, suppleness, constant renewal of skin cells, and is vital for skin elasticity. Fluoride leads to the breakdown of collagen in muscle, skin, bone, tendon, cartilage, the lungs, the kidneys, and the trachea. For example, the *Journal of the American Medical Association* and the New England Journal of Medicine have both reported greater incidence of hip fractures in fluoridated areas.[15, 16]

The National Institute of Environmental and Health Services has linked fluoridation with cancer.[17] In a 1975 survey, Dr. John Yiamouyiannis showed that people in areas with fluoridated water actually have higher incident rates of death from cancer than those in non-fluoridated areas.[18]

It was first observed as early as the 1930s that all fluoride compounds (both inorganic and organic) inhibit thyroid hormones. In fact, to reduce the activity of the thyroid gland for those suffering from over active thyroid (hyperthyroidism), many countries subsequently used numerous fluoride compounds as treatment.

How does fluoride do all this? Yiamouyiannis explains, "Fluoride interacts with the bonds which maintain the normal shape of proteins," he continues. "With distorted protein, the immune system attacks its own protein—the body's own tissue."[19] In simpler terms, fluoride causes a precarious confusion in your immune system, causing it to attack the body's own tissues, and in doing so, increases the tumor growth rate in those people who are cancer prone. Further, fluoride inhibits antibody formation in the bloodstream. *Do you need any more reasons to be cautious in using fluoride?*

Avoiding stimulants, sedatives, and drugs, such as caffeine and nicotine, and reducing alcohol intake is next on the list. Remember, coffee and black tea have high caffeine levels and act as diuretics in your body. How many of us have had a sudden sense of urgency for a bathroom break after having had a cup of tea? Green tea has cancer-fighting properties, but it also contains fluoride, so it should be limited in its use. Rooibos or nettle leaf teas are the better alternatives, or drink water (eight, 8 oz. glasses daily). It's best to drink purified or filtered water to avoid known toxins and heavy metals in tap water. Distilled water is another great source of refreshment (you can add trace minerals and/or a pinch of sea salt to replenish it). A prevalent myth is that distilled water leeches minerals from the body. Nope. First of all, minerals that are part of your cells cannot simply be leeched out by distilled water or any other variety of water.

Secondly, the amount of minerals you absorb from water are insignificant to the actual nutrient requirements of your body. You get the bulk of your minerals through those wonderful raw veggies. That whole photosynthesis trick that you learned about in high school allows plants to convert the inorganic minerals they absorb from soil into organic minerals that your body actually uses. Distilled water very efficiently removes contaminants, body toxins, and minerals.

There is the overt stress of navigating a traffic jam, but there is covert stress caused by poor digestion and improper eating habits. Basically, just give your body the best fuel possible to work with, whenever you can. Removing toxins and learning how to optimize your eating habits will be essential for creating peak health, reduced stress, and increased well-being. *But every body is different.* Depending on your symptoms, genetic predispositions, or environmental exposures, you may do better with different levels of nutrients and types of food than someone else.

Listen to your body. *Tune in.* Instead of eating the same foods habitually, treat yourself to exploring new flavors and have new colors on your plate. *Play with your food!* Eating should be an experience, not merely a routine. You're here, so why not find enjoyment in every single experience that you have?

Plus, don't think you have to be completely perfect with your diet. It's great if we can all eat well 80 to 95 percent of the time. If you do that your body usually has a pretty good reserve to compensate for any insult you might cause by, say, eating potato salad with heavy mayo and grilled meat at a great neighborhood barbecue! The exception here is that if you really are sick, then you'll want to get as close to 100 percent perfection with your diet as possible to improve your opportunities for recovery.

Now you can easily see why adopting a positive approach to healthy eating is equally about adopting a healthy approach to life. For too long we've treated our bodies with so little regard. The additional stress of poor eating habits that we put on our bodies translates into subliminal mental stress as our body struggles to cope. Yet, for all of our mal-treatment, it continues to do all that it can to keep functioning seamlessly. Healthy eating is about great food choices, and it's also about slowing down—it's about chewing your food and being aware of what you eat and how you feel when you're eating. This requires more Being. Relax while eating and taste your food. Be present. Be sensitive to your body's needs, truly care for yourself, and nurture your own Being by knowing what will nourish you.

Bon appetite!

5

Hey, where are you going? You don't have to change into special clothes or clear the furniture out of the middle of the floor. We're going to start right where you are!

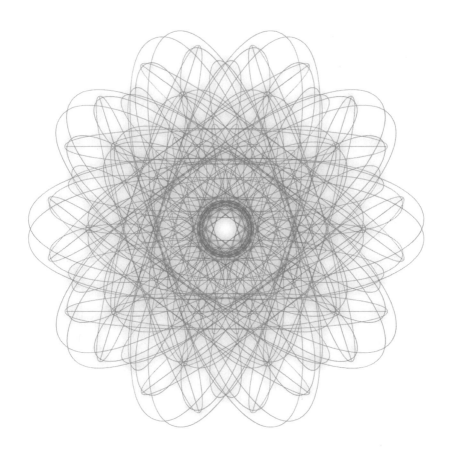

Stretching

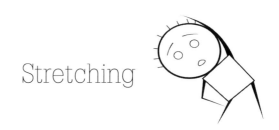

Ever watch a cat stretch? They just instinctively seem to lengthen every muscle fiber to its fullest, releasing tension with such a peaceful contentment. We're gonna borrow a little of that.

How can you expect to relax when your muscles are holding on to so much tension? We walk around so tense that it actually begins to feel natural. We all tend to hold stress in different parts of our body (neck, shoulders, lower back). Are you carrying one too many items in your favorite bag, causing neck, shoulder, or back pain? Do you need to adjust your seat height at work or in your car to unburden your knees? Or do you start to get a twinge every time a certain someone calls?

Where, when, and why you hold tension in specific areas of your body can be a revealing clue as to both your internal mental workings and external stressors (both physical and emotional). If you listen, the tension in your body can actually put you in touch with certain life issues that you need to pay closer attention to.

Using the Stop Technique from Chapter 4 will help you to become more aware of the sensations in your body and when you need to release some tightness. Stretching is such a simple, easily available, and relaxing activity, that we typically forget to use.

When you stretch, you also improve your flexibility. Flexibility is defined as the range of motion available to your joint or joints. It not only improves muscle balance around a joint, it also improves your posture.

You already know that stretching realigns your muscle fibers—getting those kinks and knots out—and allows your circulation to once again flow freely throughout your body in an even and balanced way. Better blood circulation will also bring nutrients to your cells and remove waste byproducts. The overall feeling of relaxation brings you a natural sense of well-being and relief from tension.

Beyond relaxation, it's especially important before and after exercise. Some people neglect to do it at the end of an exercise session, but it actually speeds up your recovery process. Most people aren't aware of it, but whenever your muscles perform exercise, they tighten and shorten as a result. So, stretching them out helps to restore their length. When those muscle fibers are intertwined, scar tissue requires more time to heal.

Studies have proven conclusively that performing stretching exercises reduces your risk of injury and soreness. How? It increases not only the blood and nutrient supply to help maintain your muscles and cartilage, but it also reduces the soreness you feel the next day by decreasing the build-up of lactic acid in your muscles.

Listen to your body and be gentle when stretching. Avoid stretching your muscles to the point of actual pain. You should stretch only to the point of minimal discomfort.

Never start your workout with stretching! The American Council on Exercise points out that you should never stretch cold muscles. A slight warm-up session—enough to make you start a slight sweat and to breathe heavier—is what you need before stretching. Here is a list of when not to stretch:

» Following a recent fracture.
» When your joints or muscles are hurt, infected, or in any way inflamed.
» After muscle strains or ligament sprains.
» Whenever sharp pains are felt in your joints or muscles.[1]

Let's talk about some ways to loosen up! You don't have to change into special clothes or clear the furniture out of the middle of the floor. We over-complicate so many things. We're going to start right where you are.

Simple Stretching Technique

(adapted from Edmund Jacobson[2])

We're going to add in a little method called autogenics to help tell your body how to relax. Start simply by gently leaning back in your chair. With both feet flat on the floor, get comfortable. Rest your hands comfortably in your lap.

» Let's begin by stretching your legs out in front of you as far as they can go. Relax for a few seconds and then repeat this.

» With your legs outstretched, move your toes toward you with heels out, hold...turn your toes back down away from you... hold...relax. Let go.

» Now, tighten the muscles in your calves and those in your thighs. Tight. Hold it, hold it...and relax.

» Bring your legs back down slowly to their original position and relax all the muscles in your feet, all the muscles in your calves, and all the muscles in your thighs. Let your legs feel lose, limp, and relaxed.

» Focus and feel that wonderful relaxation coming up from your toes, up your calves, and your thighs. Feeling nicely relaxed, be calm...and...very relaxed. Calm and relaxed. Enjoy the relaxation. Commit the sensation to memory.

» Now, move your arms out to the sides. Make two fists and tighten the muscles in your fingers. Feel the tightness...hold it, hold it... and relax. Let your arms go down to their resting position. Feel that relaxation. Now stretch your arms again. Tighten the muscles in your wrists, in your forearms, in your upper arms...hold it, hold it...let go, just let go, let your arms go down to their original position. Stop for a second and take your time to really notice that quieting feeling of relaxation through your fingers, hands, forearms, and upper arms. Let your arms go completely loose and limp. Take your time to increase that feeling of relaxation—very relaxed, very calm, very relaxed and calm.

» Next, arch your back backward, pull your shoulders in, and raise your chest. Tighten the muscles in your chest, your abdomen, your back, and your neck. Hold it...hold it...let go of the tension. Just let go of the tension. Notice your muscle relaxation. Take time to feel the muscles relax in your chest, in your abdomen, in your neck, and across your back. All your muscles feel lose, limp, and relaxed.

» Now, tighten the muscles in your face—first the muscles around your forehead, then the muscles around your eyes. Make them tighter. Hold it...hold it...and relax. Now, tighten the muscles of your cheeks, the muscles around your mouth, and the muscles of your chin. Make them tighter...hold it, hold it...and relax. Let all the muscles in your face relax, first the muscles of your chin, then the muscles around your mouth, the muscles of your cheeks, the muscles around your eyes, the muscles of your forehead. Let all the tension drain from your face. Let your jaw sag. Take your time to enjoy the feeling of relaxation. Very relaxed and very calm. Relaxed and calm. Commit this sensation to memory.

» Now, breathe in through your nose, slowly and deeply. Breathe the air down into your abdomen. Hold it, hold it...and slowly breathe out through your nose. Feel the relaxation. Breathe in, tense up...breathe out and release all tension. Easy.

» Once again, take a very deep breath, hold it...hold it and slowly release it and with it let go of all pressure, your frustrations, your anxieties, feeling more and more relaxed. Relaxed and peaceful.

» Now, take some time to scan your body. If you notice a tension spot, please take your time to release that tightness.

Stretching is such a simple way to relieve stress. We've become so accustomed to our tension; teach your body what it feels like to relax. Commit this sensation to memory.

There are plenty of websites on which you'll learn a variety of stretching exercises and techniques. The one most highly recommended is active isolated stretching, which you'll find uses several different postures to work your different muscle groups. Choose ones that work the best for your physicality and the particular parts of the body in which you tighten up when stressed. This can make a humongous difference in relatively short time. Oh, and stretching is *free!*

You can do it anywhere. After a busy day at work, stretches can be done discreetly at the bus stop or in your car when stopped at a traffic light. Learn even more by finding a yoga class in your area. Some are low cost or free.

Stretching

Stretching before bed is a must. By releasing muscular tension you'll rest more soundly. The increased blood flow will even bring you more energy in the morning.

This is a relatively small time investment that pays huge dividends. Breathe deeply and freely as you stretch. The focus turns to re-claiming time for your *self*.

6

Not just stress relief....
The more vital you feel, the more rarely you get sick.
Move and enjoy your body, not because you have to, but
because it makes you feel good.

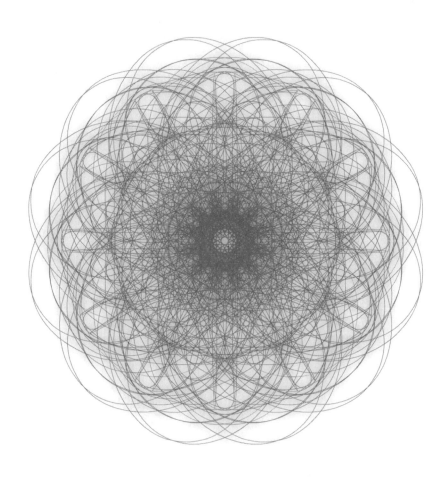

Movement

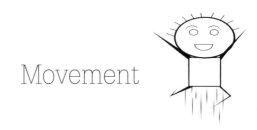

You think you know what I'm going to say. You almost passed by this chapter just to avoid the guilt you've been beating yourself up with about exercise. But I'm going to surprise you!

You see now that stress is not something that you can simply will away. It requires that you first acknowledge its presence and define both its effect and its use. Still, there is the issue of how to productively release the enormous energy and reserves that it calls upon. You've got to effectively discharge that build-up in order to reduce your cortisol levels (yes, that all-important generator of cardio-vascular issues and belly fat). You need to exercise, but here's the surprise:

Most people have been exercising *too much*! That's right! Go hug a scientist, because their research has revealed that there's a far more efficient way to keep healthy!

Just from observation, we should have known this. Ever see a llama pull up lame from running a marathon? Ever see a man-eating tiger just out for a jog? That's because animals, yes that includes you, were designed for short bursts of energy with periods of rest—not long exercise sessions or marathons.

Your body was designed for movement. There's no getting around it. Every functional system in your body requires the energy that's driven by movement. You have to exercise!

Additionally, if you're under routine stress of any kind—mental, physical, emotional—you need the release that comes through exercise.

For every pound of fat that you gain, your body will create seven miles of new blood vessels! All of this extra mileage will now require that your body work even harder to pump blood, which now puts a strain on your heart. The effects don't stop there, because this may reduce oxygenation and nutrient replenishment in other tissues. The good news is that when you lose one pound, your body will break down and re-absorb the excess vessels.

So how much exercise is recommended? After you've been cleared by your doctor, consider high-intensity interval training (HIIT) as your primary exercise. You'll do this for 20 minutes, three times a week. Yep! Twenty minutes, three times a week.

Why Is Interval Training So Effective?

1. It improves not only your fitness level, but also your ability to use oxygen. Also, you burn more calories as you increase your oxygen use.
2. Interval-training workouts will actually expand the network of blood vessels that furnish your muscles, giving you more energy. And the number of mitochondria (the energy generators in your cells) within that extra blood supply also get a tweak, thereby increasing your physical endurance.
3. Even post-exercise it increases your fat burning and calorie expenditure. Yes, that means you literally burn more calories *while you rest or sleep!*
4. It can naturally increase your human growth hormone (HGH) levels. This little addition promotes both building new muscle and consequently fat burning.

The "secret" to why HIIT is so effective is clear, according to fitness expert Phil Campbell, author of *Ready Set Go*:

Most exercise programs today are built based upon a very incomplete picture of the physiology of your body. For example, long slow cardio, "calories in, calories out," would be a perfect way to look at the body if it were all slow-twitch fiber… (but) there are three muscle fiber types: slow, fast, and super-fast…both those types of fast-twitch fibers are essentially 50 percent of your muscle fibers that don't get recruited until you add a velocity of movement.[1]

What he's saying is that, if you don't actively engage and strengthen all three muscle fiber types (and energy systems), then you're simply not going to work both processes of your heart muscle. Unfortunately, many believe that cardio exercise is building their heart muscle, but that's really not true. What they're actually working is your slow-twitch muscle fibers, yet they're still not effectively employing the very important anaerobic process of their heart.

Those fast-twitch fibers are largely glycolytic and they store a lot of glucose. That's right, good ole *sugar*. So when you use these muscles, you not only create the stimulus needed to truly produce more muscle, you also enlarge the glucose storage reservoir within your muscle, which in turn enhances your insulin sensitivity. Controlling your insulin levels is one of the most powerful ways to reduce your cancer risks. Talk about a *win-win!* This is the secret behind why one of the primary health benefits of HIIT exercise is normalizing your insulin. Conventional aerobics simply doesn't do this as efficiently.

How Are Conventional Cardio or Aerobic Exercises Different From the Anaerobic Exercise of HIIT?

Without getting too technical, while oxygen is used to break down glucose by aerobic exercise, the anaerobic exercises make use of phospho-creatine, which is stored in your muscles, for this same process. Aerobic exercises concentrate on strengthening and the muscles involved in respiration. It has been shown to improve the circulation of blood and transportation of oxygen in your body, reduce blood pressure, and burn fat.

On the other hand, anaerobic exercise helps build strength and muscle mass, stronger bones, and increases speed, power, muscle strength, and the metabolic rate as well. It concentrates on burning the calories when your body is at rest. How? HIIT increases your resting metabolic rate (RMR) in the 24 hours following high-intensity exercise. That's right! Even after you're done with your workout, more calories are burned off.

But be prepared: You will have to really work hard during your high-intensity periods to make this a fat-burning workout—perhaps harder than you're used to—hence getting checked out by your doctor *first*.

Also, to avoid injury, increase your intensity by only small increments every 7 to 10 days, but no more. If you're not someone who routinely exercises or if you have any physical issues, don't go all-out. After you're cleared by your doctor, aim for moderate exertion—just enough to raise your breathing rate. You'll still get benefits you want, but without risking injury. So, how is it done?

High-Intensity Interval Training

Ultimately here you want to exercise vigorously enough so that you reach your anaerobic threshold because this is where the "magic" happens that will trigger your growth hormone release and burn-up of belly fat!

1. 3-minute warm-up.
2. 30 seconds at full intensity (respiration increases, muscles burn, profuse sweating by your second or third repetition).
3. 90 seconds medium pace (respiration should recover).
4. Repeat steps 2 and 3 just seven times.
5. Finish with 5-minute cool-down.

Interval training can also be easily done on a recumbent bike, elliptical trainer, in-line skates, mini-trampoline, or even using squat thrusts. Treadmills are simply too slow in changing pace to be effective for this kind of work-out.

If you are not in great shape and just starting this, you may want to start with just two or three repetitions and then gradually work your way up to eight.

Note: There is absolutely no benefit to going beyond eight repetitions. I know you're thinking the more you do, the quicker you'll get into shape, but researchers at the University of Copenhagen have confirmed this in an article published by the *American Journal of Physiology*. Their research results are unique, because participants in the study belong to the large, but often overlooked, group of moderately overweight men (a population that has gradually become 40 percent of the male population in Denmark). The Faculty of Health and Medical Sciences followed 60 heavy—but healthy—Danish men. The participants in the study trained every day for three months. "On average, the men who exercised 30 minutes a day lost nearly 8 pounds in three months, while those who exercised for a whole hour only lost 6 pounds," reports Mads Rosenkilde, PhD student, Department of Biomedical Sciences.[2]

And 30 minutes of exercise training provides an extra bonus! According to Dr. Rosenkilde, "Participants exercising 30 minutes per day burned more calories than they should relative to the training program we set for them. In fact, we can see that exercising for a whole hour instead of a half does not provide any additional loss in either body weight or fat. The men who exercised the most lost too little relative to the energy they burned by running, biking, or rowing. 30 minutes of concentrated exercise give equally good results on the scale."

Even better, research has demonstrated that 20 minutes of high-intensity interval training, two to three times a week, can give you *greater* results than slow and steady conventional aerobics done five times a week. But the fact that you can improve your insulin sensitivity by nearly 25 percent with a time investment of less than *one hour a month* is no less than astounding.

Recovery Time Between Sessions Is Vital

Yep, you have to take a day off between HIIT sessions. This recovery time is crucial to allowing your body to replenish energy stores and repair damaged soft tissues (muscles, tendons, ligaments) and the removal of chemicals that build up as a result of cell activity during exercise. Exercise or any other physical work causes changes in your body such as muscle tissue breakdown and the depletion of energy stores (muscle glycogen) as well as fluid loss. Giving your body a day in between allows these stores to be replenished and allows tissue repair to occur.

Waking up at the same time every day to get your workout in helps your body to regulate many different body functions for optimal performance all day long. It also will "rev-up" your metabolism, helping you to burn more calories throughout your day. But evening exercise can be an invaluable tool for blowing-off steam and releasing the tensions of the day.

Weighty Matters

On that day off, you'll still want to do some training with light weights for about 15 minutes. This can be done twice a week just to keep your muscles toned. For this, use light free weights, resistance bands, or your own body weight to build muscular strength and endurance. When most folks think of strength training, it usually consists of weightlifting, but really you should also incorporate core body training, because new muscle tissue is produced whenever your muscle cells are required to lift something heavy on a repetitive basis. You can start small, doing a few push-ups or stretches before going to bed and learning exercises to do with resistance bands. A University of Michigan study proved that after an average of 18 to 20 weeks of progressive resistance training, an adult can add 2.42 pounds of lean muscle to their body mass and increase overall strength by 25 to 30 percent.[3]

Okay, here is a little bad news: on average, you'll lose 5 percent of your muscle mass every 10 years after the age of 35 if you don't do some sort of training. In 10 years, a person easily can lose two and a half pounds of muscle! Not good! Remember, muscle is used to burn fat, so this muscle loss results in increased difficulty in maintaining your ideal weight. You simply no longer have sufficient muscle mass to burn those wonderful calories that you consume. So, if you don't deliberately rebuild your muscle through exercise, you'll need to eat 150 to 450 fewer calories every day for 10 years to maintain your current weight. *Ouch!*

"Healthy muscle is not only about being stronger and bigger," says Miriam Nelson, director of the John Hancock Center for Physical Activity and Nutrition at Tufts University. Strength training not only builds muscle, but it helps keep older folks steady, surefooted, capable, and strong enough to do basic things like get out of a chair. She continued, "A 70-year-old active individual is probably younger from a biomarker standpoint—muscle strength, balance, body composition, blood pressure, cholesterol levels—than a 40-year-old inactive individual."[4] Her breakthrough research revealed that previously sedentary postmenopausal women who lifted weights twice a week for a year could increase their muscle strength by nearly 80 percent. *Are you motivated yet?* We're talking about a 15-minute commitment twice a week!

Maintaining muscle also requires getting an adequate amount of protein from your diet as mentioned earlier in Chapter 4. A 2009 study conducted by D. Paddon-Jones found that whether young or old, 4 ounces of lean beef, eaten immediately after a resistance training workout, boosted the body's muscle-building rate by 50 percent. He also found that eating as much as 12 ounces of beef didn't provide any extra benefits.[5] Remember, other excellent sources of protein include wild salmon, halibut, cod, lentils, black beans, walnuts, almonds, and quinoa.

Also try to mix up your exercise routine every now and then. Your brain is designed to always conserve as much energy as possible, and diversity will keep varying how much to use. Go for a walk or dance to boost your energy, mood, and cardiovascular health. Do yoga, tai-chi, or stretching to relax and improve your flexibility. In addition, try to sweat profusely at least three times a week to release toxins (try steam in your shower or use a sauna).

Exercise and What to Eat, When?

Remember, when you don't have proper nutrition, and when you don't feed yourself, it puts your body under stress to function optimally, which will contribute subliminally to any other stress you may have. So, when it comes to exercise and the questions become, "To eat or not to eat?" and "Before or after?" the answer is *both*!

Before

The research is in and it shows that exercising after short-term fasting (such as before breakfast) may increase the amount of fat you burn. On the other hand, eating a meal that stimulates a low blood glucose response prior to exercise may also boost your body's actual use of body fat (instead of glucose). Research further shows that if you exercise for longer than 60 minutes without supplying your body with any nutrients, you will actually burn *fewer* calories and even less fat than if you had eaten, and your post-exercise metabolic rate (or rate of calorie burning) is also lower.

You've got several factors to consider, including how long you exercise, your type of exercise, your exercise experience, and health factors that may play a role in how you process food. That said, you know that if you eat, you need to also allow time for that food to digest before exercising (otherwise you'll cramp). Also, you know that more time is needed before more intense activities.

» Large meal: more than 3 to 4 hours.
» Small meal: 2 to 3 hours.
» Liquid meal: 1 to 2 hours.
» Light snack: less than 1 hour.

When you consider the amount of time that it takes to digest even a light snack, you can easily conclude that the majority of the "fuel" that you'll use during most exercise is not coming from the food you have just eaten. Nope. You're using glycogen and fat that was already stored in your muscles, liver, and fat cells.

Usually, you'll have enough of that stored fuel to last for one to two hours of intense to very intense work or three to four of moderate intensity. So technically, you're covered without eating. *But*, when you don't eat at all, you then risk breaking down muscle and causing a great deal of stress to your body during exercise.

Keeping all of what we've just reviewed in mind, doesn't it just make sense to have a regular meal four hours prior to your workout, followed by a small 200-calorie snack one hour before you exercise?

Keep it light. Pre-workout you don't want to have large amounts of proteins and fats (even if they're healthy proteins and fats) because these types of fuel take a longer time to digest and will pull precious oxygen and energy-delivering blood to your stomach and away from your exercising muscles. They also carry a greater risk of giving you stomach cramps during exercise.

Choose whole foods, not sports drinks, energy bars, or powders, which will only add hazardous toxins, chemicals, useless calories, sugar, and caffeine to your diet. Hydrate with filtered water. Have at least 16 ounces two hours earlier and another 8 ounces 10 to 20 minutes right before exercise.

The amount of 200 calories may be hard to visualize, so consider:

» Raw nuts (walnuts, almonds, pistachios) (½ cup).
» Brown rice (½ cup) with black beans (½ cup).
» Banana with almond butter (2 Tbsp.).
» Multi-grain crackers (10) with hummus (3 Tbsp.).

After

Food eaten after your workout will have a huge influence on the overall health effects that your workout has on your body. You certainly don't want to have done all of that work for nothing! Your goal is not to replace every calorie that you just burned, but to give you just enough fuel so that you can maintain a high-yielding metabolism.

Remember that after you've exercised, your muscles have been broken down due to the release of hormones, and your body is also nitrogen-poor. This is when it becomes important to provide your body with the correct nutrients to stop this catabolic process that's happening in your muscles and shift the whole recycling process over toward muscle repair and growth. When you miss that window of opportunity, that entire catabolic process will go too far and can potentially damage your muscles. Amino acids from high-quality animal proteins, along with carbohydrates from vegetables (not grains), are absolutely necessary for this process.

After a workout with weights, wait 15 to 30 minutes and then have a high-quality protein and vegetable carbohydrate in order to help repair your damaged muscles. After cardio, wait 45 to 60 minutes and have a high-quality protein and vegetable-type carbohydrate. Hydrate after both with 16-ounces of an electrolyte-balanced water. Protein provides you with essential amino acids, which are the building blocks for muscle repair and growth. Based on current research, it seems that instead of just simply reducing calorie intake, eating specifically fewer carbohydrates after exercise can actually enhance your insulin sensitivity. Getting your insulin sensitivity under control is so important for maintaining good over-all health, increasing well-being, and reducing stress.

Good sources of animal protein include:

» Kefir (organic, plain).

» Eggs (organic, from pastured hens).

» Chicken (organic, humanely raised, free-range).

» Beef (organic, grass-fed).

» Whey protein (minimally processed and derived from organic, grass-fed, non-hormonally treated cows).

Remember that portion size should be limited to between 2 to 4 ounces. Favorable sources of carbohydrates include:

» All raw vegetables (especially dark green, leafy vegetables such as organic spinach, kale, or Swiss chard, but limiting carrots and beets, which are high in sugar).

» Low fructose fruits like organic lemon, limes, passion fruit, apricots, plums, cantaloupe, and raspberries. (Avoid high-fructose fruits like apples, watermelons, and pears.)

Locker Room Pep Talk

Based on data collected for the National Health and Nutrition Examination Survey (NHANES) for 2005/6 and 2009/10, restricting the amount of time that you spend seated every day to less than three hours boosts the life expectancy of adults by an extra two years, as reported in the journal BMJ Open.[6]

Exercise boosts your glutathione level, which heightens your body's own antioxidant defenses, helps boost your immune system, and improves over-all detoxification.[7] Never heard of glutathione? Most folks haven't, but here's the thing—it is by far *the* most important antioxidant as both the director of your immune system and principal detoxifier. It's sort of like Velcro—all the toxins (free-radicals and toxins like mercury and other heavy metals) stick to glutathione, which then carries them right out of your body via bile and stool. Research shows that increased glutathione levels actually decrease any muscle damage, reduce your recovery time, increase both strength and endurance, and shift your metabolism from fat production to muscle development.[8]

Ordinarily, glutathione is manufactured and recycled in your body—except when your toxic load is too high. When that happens, it can be a root cause of a multitude of issues such as autism, Alzheimer's disease, chronic fatigue syndrome, arthritis, heart disease, cancer, chronic infections, autoimmune disease, diabetes, Parkinson's disease, asthma, kidney problems, liver disease, and more.

So, the benefits of exercise are endless. Not just for your cardiovascular and immune systems; it also helps to preven, delay, and reduce the cognitive impairment that comes along with aging (or shall we just call it "maturing"?).

Did you know exercise has been proven to actually slow down the aging process? Telomeres are microscopic parts of your chromosomes that control aging. You know those little plastic caps at the end of your shoelaces? You can imagine telomeres as being a lot like that at the ends of your chromosomes. When you're young, they're longer and they gradually shorten with age. *Guess what hastens their decline?* STRESS!

Your nutrition, lifestyle, and environment all directly influence the rate at which those telomeres shorten by increasing your cortisol levels and oxidative stress. Exercise improves your telomere maintenance by increasing the activity of the enzyme telomerase, which builds and repairs your telomeres. Specifically in terms of its protection against stress, exercise protects the structure of your hippocampus and temporal lobes from all that cortisol that gets dumped in from you adrenal glands.

Another brain chemical that gets a benefit from exercise is the famous brain derived neuortrophic factor—*oh yeah, everyone's talking about that!* Let's just agree to call it BDNF while I explain that it generates brand new brain cells in your temporal lobes (the brain sector involved in your memory) and your prefrontal cortex (involved in both planning and judgment), but those new cells only last about four weeks and then die off *unless* stimulated with some fresh social interaction or new mental exercise. Yep! You have to exercise regularly in order to get this new supply *and* you have to get some mental stimulation.

Exercise also has been shown to have a very powerful impact on your psyche, and is a very potent tool if you're feeling blue, no matter what the reason. It increases your levels of endorphins and serotonin or "feel-good" hormones. When you feel good, it's definitely easier to Be—to see the silver lining and become more engaged with life and the people around you.

Trading in the Big "C" for the Big "E"

T cells, so named because they are developed in your thymus gland, are immune cells that circulate throughout your blood and lymph system. T cells also have a great nickname: natural killercells (NKs)—because they act as assassins trained to destroy damaged, cancerous, or infected cells. Laura Bilek, Graham Sharp, and Geoffrey Thiele, from the University of Nebraska Medical Center, and Daniel Shackelford, Colin Quinn, and Carole Schneider, from Rocky Mountain Cancer Rehabilitation Institute, analyzed immune cells called T cells in the blood of cancer survivors before and after a 12-week exercise program. What did they learn? A significant portion of these immune cells reverted from a mature form, which isn't very effective at combating disease, to a more youthful form, much more able to fight off cancer and infections.[9]

So by having cancer survivors exercise for several weeks after they finish chemotherapy, their immune systems actually improved and became more effective, potentially fending off future incidents of cancer! This might explain why exercise can significantly reduce the chances of secondary cancers in survivors or lessen the risks of cancer altogether in people who haven't had the disease. Are you awake now? Looking for your gym clothes?

Study leader Laura Bilek pointed out that there is already a large volume of research validating the many positive associations between exercise and cancer—notably, that exercise can diminish the risk of initiating several different types of cancers to begin with, frequently improves prognosis in cancer patients, and can decrease the risk of recurrence and secondary cancers survivors. What had been absent was the unidentified mechanism behind these phenomena. "What we're suggesting is that with exercise, you might be getting rid of T cells that aren't helpful and making room for T cells that might be helpful," Bilek says.[10]

Once you've started improving your diet, adding exercise will start to rebalance the levels of neurotransmitters in your brain, improve memory, enhance your mood, and just keep you younger. The more vital you feel, the more rarely you get sick. Move and enjoy your body, not because you have to, but because it makes you feel good!

7

The only thing we can influence (and sometimes with great difficulty) is our reaction to the changes and challenges in our environment—that's central to our health.

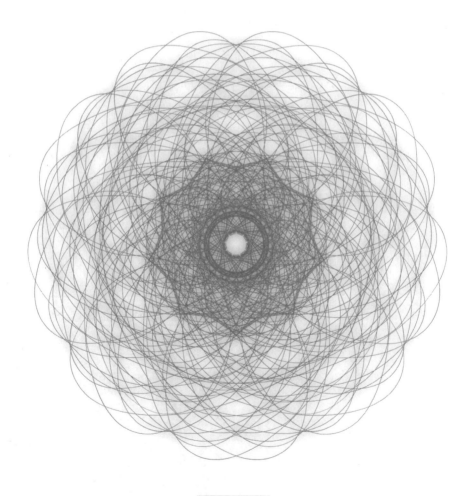

Anxiety (or Dance With the Elephants)

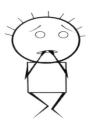

Masks, masks, masks! We spend *way* too much energy trying to ignore the elephants in our room. All of us are so attached to events and outcomes as *the* measurement for how are lives are going. If you're going through any of the items from the earlier list of "life's most stressful events," that needs to be addressed.

Why? This goes back to the earlier discussion regarding environment and the way that your thoughts, attitudes, associations, and misperceptions directly affect your health.

We tend to assume that whatever we are focused on consciously is dominant, hence the assumption that "thinking positively" or doing "affirmations" will override any negativity in our conscious awareness. But what if I told you that science believes your conscious mind controls only about 10 percent, whereas your unconscious mind represents 90 percent of your mind power. According to work done by John A. Bargh, a professor of psychology at Yale, researchers in independent studies have also shown that, once covertly triggered, an unconscious goal will persist with the same level of resolve that is raised by our conscious pursuits.[1] Your brain appears to use the very same neural circuits to execute an unconscious act as it does a conscious one. Kinda makes you wonder: "What's in my unconscious?"

As mentioned in Chapter 1, your mind is filled with childhood associations, collected family superstitions, urban myths, and inaccurate news media reporting. There's some good stuff too, but there's also a lot of limiting, self-sabotaging, habitual thought patterns, attitudes, and beliefs. It's impossible to guess how or when an unconscious drive may suddenly become conscious, or under what conditions anyone is able to override hidden urges by sheer willpower.

There are many, many programs and therapies on the market that offer personal transformation—some well-intentioned, some merely opportunistic scams. They'll promise to take you beyond your filters, hidden contexts, hidden desires, motivations, angles, personal myths, illusions, and more. But from what you know now, is dominance over your unconscious in any situation really realistic? Should that be the goal?

I'm rolling around to the point that your reactions to the stressors in your life and the way that you identify and perceive those stressors need careful examination, because all of it is being influenced outside of your immediate awareness and ALL of this is affecting not only your health but your sense of well-being.

You see it now. You have a more comprehensive view of the multitudinous crap load that you're trying to wield conscious control over. Add another person (or persons) into the mix, and you're now inviting all of their "stuff" too. Now pile onto that an actual issue, problem, or grievance that you're all trying to solve together. It truly is a miracle that any of us communicate at all or get anything done! The room is full of elephants that no one will acknowledge.

With every relationship, there are issues and growth to experience. Is it possible that starting with yourself is best? So often, people admit that they were able to improve their relationships (and work environment as well), when they stopped running away from the conflicts that they encountered in their personal lives. Our tendency is to reach the same impasse across each relationship. You hear it again and again. Someone will relate that, until they took a break, stepped back, and worked out their intimate and personal issues, they couldn't meet and be close with the "right person." The same concept holds true for any kind of relationship. Sometimes we have to take a deep breath, turn the mirror around, and determine if there are some changes we need to make.

Perfection

A myth—whose quest causes anxiety. Let it go.

Mistakes

You screwed up! There, I said it. Acknowledgment is your first step. Note, I did not say that *you* were a screw-up! Big difference. You've made mistakes, and if you're very, very lucky you'll make many more. *Congratulations!*

Anxiety (or Dance With the Elephants)

It means that you're alive—a living, breathing person on planet Earth. Recognize too that there is a huge difference between a mistake and just plain misbehavior, which for simplicity's sake we'll define just as improper conduct, rudeness, or wrong-doing without cause or consciousness. We all know some highly evolved people who simply behave badly and there's no "mistake" to it. What we're speaking about in this segment is having made an unfortunate choice.

Nothing brings on the anxiety like a "fork in the road" or its consequences. Albert Einstein is credited with saying, "Anyone who has never made a mistake has never tried anything new." However, the most self-devaluing part of making mistakes is not the mistake, but how you interpret the error (*perception*). Remember from Chapter 1 our discussion about the cascade of biochemical signals that flow through your body based on your reactions to your environment? Mistakes can cause gigantic reactions.

Obviously there are some mistakes, tragic mistakes, which are more significant than others, but they too are a part of life. In the words of Friedrich Nietzsche, "That which does not kill us makes us stronger."

Anxiety over making mistakes can translate into either a fear of failure or a fear of success. Ultimately what happens *next* is the core of the experience and where your *STRESS* lies. Consequence—the unknown void that follows failure (or success)—can certainly be problematic. But you've made mistakes and *you're still here*!

You are a born problem-solver. Every day you deal with problems and mistakes caused by you and others (small, large, tiny, medium). You do it all day long. It's second nature to you, but you don't give yourself credit. Most of the time you just let it go. When you can easily spot a problem and redirect before the consequences are felt, you feel great. Homerun! But when you really miss the ball and it barely leaves the plate, that's when the inner critic comes out and that's when you really have to keep an eye on your reaction to the error.

Blame is usually our immediate response. Some will assume all the blame themselves, which avoids a possible messy confrontation or may give them a false sense of control over the possibility of a repeat (if it was just their mistake, then they can make sure it doesn't happen again).

Others will blame anyone but themselves. Then there are those who will blithely act as if nothing happened and merely wait for the fallout (often hoping, wishing, and praying that it will all just go away). Also, there's the justified approach wherein the person believes "I *had* to do that because so-and-so did such-and-such," or "Anyone would have done the same thing if they were in my shoes." Lastly, there's the person who believes that everything in life is happening *to* them—outside forces beyond their control have caused all of the wrongs in their life. We've all engaged in each of these scenarios at one time or another, to greater or lesser degree. Even our basic need to control events and outcomes can unintentionally twist our most sincere efforts. So, maybe assigning blame is not the most helpful route toward resolution of the mistake.

Accountability, however, is valuable and a necessity often overlooked (or avoided). *What's the difference between blame and accountability?*

Blame seeks to condemn and punish, while accountability focuses on what happened and what needs to be improved. That said, making an apology should never be used as a defensive tactic merely to gain acceptance, recognition, approval, affirmation, or some other angle. Acknowledging your part in an offense is not just a sign of maturity, it allows much needed movement forward (growth).

Accountability will not undo the harmful past actions, although if done sincerely it can undo some of the negative emotional effects left in the wake of those actions for you both. Not being accountable leaves you wide open for esteem-robbing, self-reproach, and guilt. But know what you're apologizing *for*. Step back and look into it more deeply.

Maya Angelou said, "When you know better, you do better,"[2] and this is certainly something to aspire to, but not always true. There are times when you *know* better, yet continue to do the same darn thing—like a moth to the flame. There's an often repeated saying, "Insanity is doing the same thing over and over again and expecting a different result." Sometimes the same issue has arisen, but in a different disguise. At other times you may blatantly just make the exact same mistake *again!* What's wrong with you? Absolutely nothing. Your actions, however, deserve some closer examination.

Anxiety (or Dance With the Elephants)

There's something about this particular life lesson that you have not taken the time to honestly explore (operative word is "honestly")—some aspect that continues to draw you in and you're acting on it. Perhaps it's some unresolved parental issue that shows up now with a significant other, a cross reprimand from a long-ago teacher revisited now with your boss, the need to compete with a peer for reward—any number of unconscious longings and unfinished business. In other words, maybe you're co-mingling some recyclables from your past with your present. But if you open up to learning from your mistakes, you will be able to move on rather than wallowing in regret or disappointment. Unless wallowing in self-pity is actually your goal—even unconsciously.

Self-pity is addictive, self-perpetuating, and carries a certain amount of power. First, it's an escape of sorts. This level of self-absorption feels good, it allows for complete mental obsession, and it also effectively separates you from reality. The bonus being that personal responsibility also gets jettisoned through self-pity.

Also, people become blinded when wrapped-up in self-pity. They genuinely can't see that they're being self-centered. Their focus is all about me, me, me. The world is constantly happening *to* them. They perpetually continue to play the victim role in their own movie. Ironically, it's also empowering because along with their Oscar award, they become entitled to demand that everyone around them feed into this distorted pity reality as well. Anxiety and depression play huge roles here too.

So, how do you break a self-pity cycle? Every day you must strive to increase your awareness so that you can begin to identify when you're slipping into self-pity mode. This initually requires a bit of effort and practice. But when you do it for a few days, it will become second nature to you.

Focus also on gratitude for even the small things in your life. Actually, that's something we all should make a daily habit. Gratitude not just for the big ticket items, but those small moments, when you look for them, can bring you a real sense of joy. You can do this for yourself *all day long*.

Regret from mistakes becomes harmful because you grow attached to that image of how you wanted things to turn out before the error. It's a natural reaction; once it has happened, you keep looping back to how things should have gone.

Now, take a closer look at that picture you're holding onto of what might have been. Find within it those elements that truly matter to you. Distinguish from the specifics of the error that happened, such as how you still want to feel, how you really want to express yourself, where you want to be, and how you want to see the world. Then get into action. Get moving with positive new ways to get there. Begin with just that feeling that you originally wanted to feel and now move toward that feeling.

Note: Actual addiction to unhealthy behaviors or substances will require more in-depth assistance from a professional source. These aren't ordinary mistakes, but signs of more serious issues to be discussed with a trained counselor or licensed therapist.

But for most people, mistakes, though painful, signal a good time for pulling off the road and taking some time for reflection. Even if the mistake was not entirely your own, it still must be dealt with and there's valuable information in it—for *you*. It is well worth it to address the elephant in the room.

Many of us were basically never taught how to sit down with a decision that needs to be made and reason it out. It's a life skill. Many mistakes are made because no time was taken for obtaining, culling, and processing information, weighing pros and cons, and creating a roadmap first to determine the best route for where you're heading.

Cut yourself some slack. Don't identify yourself with the mistake, but do try to pinpoint the error itself. What led up to the point where your blunder happened? Reevaluate your approach. Did you have so many balls in the air that you couldn't keep them prioritized? Were you rushed? Maybe it's an area where you're deficient. Did you need more information, additional knowledge, or training? Take some time to consider what you are doing, why you are doing it, how you feel, and how you make others feel. What was the reward that you were seeking? Can you really be honest (without taking on added guilt) and just identify what your true motive was from the outset on that particular road?

Nine times out of 10, you did "that thing you did" because you ultimately thought it would make things better or make you (or someone else) "happier." That's not a bad thing, but maybe a misdirected thing. Maybe, just maybe, you were attempting to gain happiness along the wrong road. Now you are on a new road and must deal with the resulting change.

The true value is found in what you do next and what you want to feel now in this moment.

Change: Facing the Crossroad Without Fear

One of the most consistent causes of anxiety is "change"—one that's happened, one that's happening, and one that's about to happen. That earlier list of stressful events says it all. Upheaval causes unrest. Change tends to include loss on some level. It's especially disruptive when it's unexpected.

Again, you are not alone here. Our innate desire for stability is natural. We simply feel more comfortable with familiar people, places, ideas, and situations than we do with unfamiliar ones. Change can feel foreign, even dangerous. Change outright demands that we become more flexible, which is not a quality commonly cultivated. It's a glaring reminder that we don't control the universe. Change comes along and demonstrates that you can't even control everything within your own little sphere of influence. You can influence things, but many things are simply out of your control. Why do we always think that we can control everything? Change comes—ready or not. Flexibility should be taught as a life skill.

Using the Stop Technique will help you to get in touch with your frustration and abate it bit by bit. Try to get perspective after you breathe. Once you've really had a chance to recognize the change and some of its layered effects, try disassembling it, breaking it down into pieces, and addressing the easier parts first. If your work problems are easier to accept than your frustrations at home, for example, then start with work and even break those work issues down into smaller pieces. You don't have to tackle everything at once.

List out for yourself which of your personal strong points can be used to help this situation. *What's that?* You say you don't know what your personal strong points are? Okay. Scratch that list for a moment. By the way, you are not alone in this. Most people cannot list five of their attributes. So sit down, dismiss your inner critic from the room, and list your personal strong points. You can by saying "I knot the top of my garbage really well before tossing it," or "I have mastered the music playlists in my car—heads always turn when I stop at a light," or "I am someone who people can trust."

You see, your anxiety is only heightened when you don't recognize what tools you've already got in your personal toolbox to deal with what you're facing. Once you've established a baseline for your personal attributes, take some time to consider which of these might be used to help you to better adapt to the new changes in your life. Now, reflect on other resources that you might be able to call on through friends or colleagues. Find reassurance in the fact that you've gotten through other changes in the past and, no matter how challenged you may seem presently, you will get through this too.

Most people have an initial negative response to change. We seem to just automatically deconstruct a new situation, seeking anything that is not quite right or to our benefit.

On the other hand, sometimes changes are eagerly anticipated— welcomed even. Here again, these too are frequently followed by a period of disappointment and regret, like "buyer's remorse" when you make a major purchase.

Now here's the big one! It becomes necessary to let go of how you think things should be and "Be" where they are. It's our resistance to change that causes anxiety. But remember, change is generally a gradual process, and so should be your movement toward accepting it. Your feet were on a particular path and now the very ground beneath you has shifted and you are required to respond or react; could you simply accept it and move forward, open to new ways to find balance in this new condition? Octavia Butler said: "Everything we touch, we change; everything we change, changes us; the only lasting truth is change."[3]

Looping Thoughts?

We are all susceptible to something called "looping thoughts." Athletes and performers often repeat positive phrases, hum a song, or chant to keep unwanted thoughts at bay during critical moments. It would do them no good in the middle of play to suddenly recall that missed pass, the bad landing, that failed block, or the overshot ball.

If worry seems impossible to decrease in your life, then let's put some boundaries on it. Experts say that there are two kinds of worrying: "current worry," which is responsive, resourceful, and productive, or "conceptual worry," which is mostly hypothetical and detrimental. Conceptual worry is about situations of which you have almost no control ("Will the pilot be able to land the plane?"), so there is very little, if anything, that you can do. This can also arise when you don't trust yourself to harness and control the demands of life, trust your ability to amass resources, or trust others around you to help you overcome your shortcomings. Although productive worry will lead you to seek a trial solution to problems, non-productive worrying often stalls out while seeking to blame or condemn. (What's she gonna do when she finds out ___? What will they think of me?)

Believe it or not, at the base of all those looping thoughts and your "inner critic" is a positive intent, though it may not seem like it when you can't shut the darn things off. They're your early warning detection system and they've been set off by something that your unconscious has held onto—a bad experience, childhood associations, family superstitions, urban myths, or something from the news.

Your temptation will be to try to simply ignore their interruptions and just get on with whatever you're doing. *How's that working out?* Yep, elephants carelessly clomping around your brain using up your energy as you try to deny their presence.

A better option is to actually pause and listen to the loop (or critic) for a moment and try to figure out what its underlying message is. Remember, its goal is to protect you. So your inquiry should begin with "What's this trying to protect me from?" Now you can consciously determine whether that protection is truly needed at all or whether some other kind of solution makes more sense. Sometimes the alert is a genuine problem. You may have overlooked an important facet of a problem area that you really do need to address. At other times, you may conclude that the whole warning is completely baseless.

The important thing is to stop and examine the root. Once again, make note of what's in your tool kit that will address the underlying concern. Which of your attributes will assist? Do you have allies with other resources? Is there a solution already in place or in progress? In this way, you're addressing the loop, the inner critic, and the worry head-on instead of leaving the elephant standing in the middle of the room.

The only thing we can influence (and sometimes with great difficulty) is our reaction to the changes and challenges in our environment, which is central to our health. Reframing your stress and anxiety toward something positive is key. As often as possible, when you notice the negativity creeping in (that sense of futility, loss, frustration, and so on) shift your awareness back to what you really *want* to feel and move toward that feeling. Again, much like being in your car on a slippery road and you're trying to regain control. You need to keep your eyes on where you want to be and keep steering toward it.

Mosh Pit Etiquette

Relationships—just like any other living thing—require care, nourishment, and maintenance. Neglect in any of these areas (whether on the acceptance or delivery end) will cause conflict.

Generally speaking, avoid quick, knee-jerk reactions (because you really can't accurately say what pulled the strings of that knee, can you?) Avoid the blame game, victim game, and the name game. Remember, louder does not mean clearer. Most of us get into trouble because of the way we communicate both our thoughts and the judgments we make (both for others and for ourselves). When we say things out of anger to hurt others, whether intentional or not (as we may feel hurt), we then escalate the situation into a war of words and feelings. That's not a healing place. It creates separation and shuts people down. Also, avoid the temptation to simply react and vent.

Anxiety (or Dance With the Elephants)

Learning to "fair fight" with a loved one (or anyone) is one thing, but being able to really *prevent* confusions and altercations is always best. Disputes resolve in one of two ways: first, solutions are found to the dispute—usually involving compromise (hopefully mutual), or second, reframing of the dispute so that it becomes neutral, that is, total and unconditional pardon of the offense in some way.

Now, does this mean that you are never going to allow yourself to get angry again? There's no getting around the fact that you may "go there." The point is not to stay "there." Try to recognize that you're there, get yourself away from there, and do some things to immediately release some of the chemicals and toxins your body has just released in response to being there. Try very hard to bring yourself back to what you really want to feel—letting go of the negative feeling. Without analyzing or judging, just try to let it go.

More graphically, just because you go "there" doesn't mean you have to get a motel room "there," order up a heap of junk food from room service, and lay around watching Pay-Per-View reruns of all the "should've said," "would've said," and "can't believe they said"—classic moment from your dispute or the next few days.

You need to be clear. If possible, take a walk or remove yourself from the situation. Make use of the Stop Technique. Now ask: What do you want in the situation? What are you feeling? What do you want to feel? What can you do to get to that feeling now? Now move toward that feeling. From this more relaxed, peaceful, happier you, re-examine the issue. Try to see it from a distanced, fly-on-the-wall perspective. Bearing in mind the truckload of subliminal influences impairing you, can you fairly consider both sides of the issue and find a compromise that may suit both? This is of course based on the ideal that life tends to be a bit messier than that. It may not always work, but this is a good technique to start with.

Sometimes a situation is beyond repair. Any resistance or dispute that separates you from your joy must be severely limited or completely eliminated.

Note: Physical or mental abuse requires complete departure—this is non-negotiable.

So, between the unwanted items slipping in from your unconscious, seemingly random change happening in your life, and relationships with their own dispositions, how do you possibly get a handle on all of that?

There are some great tools that you can access, such as reflection, meditation, prayer, the emotional freedom technique, psychological counseling, and clinical hypnosis.

Mitigation

Attentiveness and Intention: Your first line of empowerment is Being in the present moment—not what just happened or what you want to happen or expected to happen. Use the Stop Technique. What do you want to feel in this moment? Now do your best to let go of any nagging thought or negativity, and move (sometimes with great effort) toward that feeling. Make your intent to feel *that* feeling now. The more you practice, the easier it gets.

Write It Out: Write down your deepest feelings about an emotional upheaval in your life for 15 or 20 minutes a day for four consecutive days. This simple technique has been shown to provide amazing results in reduction of anxiety and emotional response as well as improved immune system functions.

Why? It gets into the left-brain/right-brain coordination aspect, but basically when you translate your experience into language, you essentially make that experience graspable. Dr. James W. Pennebaker, professor in the Department of Psychology at the University of Texas at Austin and author of several books, has concluded in his research findings that "It wasn't even necessary for people to tell their secrets to someone else. The act of simply writing about those secrets, even if they destroyed the writing immediately afterward, had a positive effect on health."[4]

Continue from there. Write a list of your other issues and know that healing can take place on many levels and may take time. Give it that space and know that change often goes slowly. Have patience, and take some time to organize your thoughts and feelings. Write a little every night. Release.

Inner Scream: Yep! Let it rip—*in your head!* Yell full blast at your boss, your kids, your spouse, the bills, the bank, the kid that does your lawn, the computer—anyone and everyone who has done something stupid or annoying. We're going to add a physical component to it, allowing your body to also release some of its pent-up energy. So while you're yelling, try adding one of these to it (unless you have shoulder issues):

» **Wall Push-Up:** Stand about 3 feet in front of a wall (or at a comfortable distance for your physical capabilities), with your feet shoulder's width apart. Outstretch your arms and place your hands flat against the wall. Lean your body toward the wall, letting the elbows bend. Push your body back with your hands until you are once again in a standing position. Let the rant commence (in your head of course).

» **Downward Dog:** This is a standard yoga position. Start on the floor in the push-up position but walk your feet toward your hands, leaving your "bum" pointing in the air, until your body looks like an upside down V. Have the heels hip-width apart and the legs straight. Push through your heels and up through your tailbone in opposing directions. The top of your head can be pointing down toward the floor or in line with the direction of force through your arms. Raise your navel upward toward your chest. This will straighten your lower back. (Yell to your heart's content—all language is acceptable. Go for it!)

When you hold onto emotions and don't express yourself, these energies create turmoil, conflict, and dis-ease in your body. Yep, *STRESS!* It's the emotional context of your worries that you need to give release to. Then you can see them more clearly for what they are and where *you* are. Then you can begin to let go. Poet Ralph Waldo Emerson said, "Nothing can bring you peace but yourself."

"If Only...Is Now" Activity

Each of us is inwardly holding onto a powerful private desire. "If only...then everything would be perfect, and I could finally relax and be happy." We all do it. This gives you a sense of direction, a goal. In our minds we set up an expectation, which can unfortunately also become a prerequisite or road block. In other words, now without that—whatever it is—we can't really and truly be happy, because it's always out there taunting you. Now when something goes well in your life, you don't fully appreciate it because, well, your ideal—whatever it is—is still out there unaccomplished or unattained. Guess what this causes? Just a little hidden anxiety. Let's relieve some of that.

Turn off your phone. Sit comfortably back in your chair, have both feet on the ground, shoulder-width apart. Start by recognizing your old friend "amazing possibility." What's this thing in your life that you can't wait to happen or never believe is going to happen? What will send you beyond happiness and over the moon?

Now, relax your arms. Really feel them just go loose, limp, and relaxed. Feel the shoulders droop slightly, your forearms getting heavy, and a sort of warmth throughout your arms. Take your time. Get really comfortable with this lack of tension and let it spread throughout your body. Feels wonderful, doesn't it?

Here you're safe, calm, and at ease. So, what will it feel like when your "If only..." happens? Maybe there are a few things that have to come together for your "If only..." When they align, what will you feel? What's your expectation? When you anticipate the emotion that will come along with it, what will you feel?

Feel it NOW! Right NOW! Let it loose! Feel the exhilaration! From the crown of your head to the bottoms of your feet, conjure up the emotion *now* and just enjoy both the release and the unbridled joy of the moment! Feel that! Give that gift to yourself NOW!

Sit and enjoy this sensation for as long as you like. Go here as often as you like. Enjoy the Joy.

Do you get it? It's always there. You do not have to wait for your life to be perfect! Spoiler alert: Glenda the Good Witch deserved a bucket of ice-cold water herself for having let Dorothy go through all of these trials only to reveal "You could have gone home at any time." Really? Splash!

When you do this, your brain reacts instantaneously by triggering reductions in stress hormones such as cortisol and epinephrine. It also releases endorphins that can relieve some physical pain *and* boosts the number of antibody-producing cells and enhances the effectiveness of

T-cells, leading to a stronger immune system. You see, your brain does not know or care whether the emotion that you're offering is in response to something you are living right now and observing, or in response to something you are imagining. It reacts only to your *perception*. Again we return to the point made in Chapter 1.

Walking the Plank

Your hands suddenly get cold and numb; all of your movements feel mechanical; you have a knot in your stomach or tightness across your neck and back; you're sweating bullets; everything you rehearsed has flown out of your head; your mouth feels like cotton; you can't seem to take a deep breath—you are experiencing one of the **6 Big Ones.**

1. Performance Anxiety

Note: *You are not the first person on Earth to encounter this dilemma.* Job interviews, giving speeches or presentations, auditions, and stage perfor-mances all share the same potential, which begs the question: How does one walk the plank, in full view of all eyes, teetering above an angry sea full of hungry alligators while maintaining a certain lightness of foot and grace under pressure? There are no reported deaths from "stage fright." Your symptoms, however annoying, will not keep you from giving an excellent presentation, but the stress response also isn't doing your body any favors and it's far from fun. This is like a herd of elephants (all your self-doubts and fears) stampeding forward.

Now let's make this adrenaline rush work for you, instead of against you. Think for a moment. This effect is really no different than what happens when you are riding a roller coaster and it takes one of those curves. The only difference is in your *perception*! You've learned to associ-ate "fright" with performance and "fun" with being on a roller coaster. How can you change this association?

» Your audience doesn't know you're having an anxiety attack de-spite the "deer in headlights" expression you now fear must be clearly displayed all across your face. They have no clue!

» Your audience is just there waiting and pretty much thinking about other things entirely (how uncomfortable their stomach feels after that meal; something they need to do at home or just did; something they heard on the news or a bill that needs to be paid).

» You might actually consider enjoying yourself! The more you enjoy yourself, the more the audience will. The more confidence you display, the more they will believe.

» Let's assume you've done your prep work. Then you will not need to do any extreme all-night rehearsal or re-writing sessions the day before. You know the piece and just need to do slow, relaxed practice to remind yourself of the ideas that you want to convey. Great!

Mitigation

Should symptoms show up, let's disarm the alarm!

» **Release Some Energy.** Walk quickly around the building a couple of times if you can. Also, you can try push-ups, sit-ups, jumping jacks, or squat-thrusts. This will not only reduce stress, it will help alleviate large muscle knots and contractions, *and* it also produces endorphins to help you actually feel better. If you're stuck in a seated position, grab the seat on both sides and pull up as hard as you can to reduce some of that flood of adrenaline.

» **Breathing Exercises.** (See Chapter 3.) By using deep breathing, your oxygen/carbon dioxide balance will be restored. Meanwhile, your body interprets this deep breath as a sort-of "danger-free" signal. So, as your stress level begins to decline, the rest of your physical symptoms will as well.

» **Laugh.** Yep! Even fake laughter will help you to relax. Remember, your brain cannot tell the difference. The enjoyment signal turns down the warning signals you're broadcasting to your adrenals, which brings your cortex back on line.

» **Hydrate** well the day before and for up to 1 hour prior to your actual performance.

» **Eat.** Nerves crank-up the adrenaline. Remember, under stress, your body will use up its sugar reserves (in preparation for you sprint away from the man-eating tiger), but you will not feel the normal hunger pangs. You probably won't even want to eat—the thought of food might make you "nauseous"—but, you will still feel the effects of low blood sugar, which are nearly identical to those of "performance anxiety": irritability, anxiety, lack of concentration, depression, forgetfulness, confusion, headache, body tremors, and cold hands and feet. Have a couple of handfuls of raw nuts, a banana, or an apple. Avoid dairy, which causes phlegm.

2. Job Interview

As much as possible, it should feel more like a conversation—not a collection of pre-fab statements and rote answers. Remember that you are interviewing potential employers as much as they are interviewing you. This is a two-way stress. Ask yourself: Is this a good fit for me here? What looks good on paper may not be what it appears for either of you. If you prepare, you are more likely to loosen up and perform better in an interview and this will reduce your stress.

» **Research.** Don't walk in cold. Learn as much as you can about the company where you hope to work. Prepare thoughts about that particular business and industry for potential interview questioning.

» **Elevator Pitch.** Have a simple 45-second statement prepared about who you are and what qualifications you have that make you perfect for that position. As you speak, *know* that you've got the job. Feel it!

» **Practice.** Grab a friend, spouse, partner, roommate, or neighbor who will give you some time and have them interview you a few days earlier and again the night before. Get their feedback and have them question you on the tough items repeatedly in various ways until you feel more solid.

» **Arrival.** Get there early. Take this time to settle in, do some breathing, and get into your mental zone. Chat up the staff if you can (just to get yourself going and maybe gain a little reconnaissance in the process).

» **Performance.** Leave your inner critic outside the building—time to go into the character of Best Employee Ever! This may sound crazy, but this is every bit a performance—have fun with it if you can. They want to know if you fit into their culture. They need to feel comfortable with you, so *you* need to feel comfortable with you. In your head, switch it around so that the interview is about them, not about you. They need to tell you what they're looking for and you need to agree that you are every bit of that *and more*. You want to project that you're a confident (not cocky), competent team player, enthusiastic (not psycho perky), and ready to get started.

> » Dress the part. The right clothing helps type-cast your character.
>
> » Your body language is vital. Consider your posture and expressions.
>
> » Make eye contact confidently (this doesn't mean stare them down). This declares to them that you're listening patiently and are self-assured in your answers to questions.
>
> » When asked a question, always find a way to highlight your positive attributes and strengths. Listen, listen, listen carefully to the interviewer, and be certain that you're answering just the question asked. Don't offer too much additional info.
>
> » Speak clearly and at a moderate, calm pace. Breathe! They need somebody to fill their position, and you are going to be really good at it!
>
> » Now pat yourself on the back! Only a small percentage of people get this far in the employment process. So give yourself credit for putting yourself on the line, even though it was difficult. Believe that a job will come through when it is the right offer and the right fit for both the company and you.

3. Audition

Auditions are very similar to job interviews, but there are a few notable differences to contemplate.

First, take a moment to seriously consider just what you can and can't control about the auditioning process. Actually commit these items to paper. Now stop beating yourself up over the things that you can't possibly control and seriously own what you can. Treat the audition process as a creative project, *your* project—with skills and habits that you can learn and get better at. Practice auditioning! Now, let's talk about that list of things that you CAN control.

This is not a firing squad, though it may feel like it, so enter the audition room confidently and be gracious and warm as you introduce yourself. This is YOUR room now. Show that you're glad to meet the people in the room (without actually gushing). Breathe. You want to project that you are well-grounded and excited about your work—even if you're desperate for the job.

When the audition is over, don't just bolt from the room. Regardless of the atmosphere or your nerves, show them what you're like under pressure and what kind of attitude they can expect from you during an actual production. Your exit should *always* be warm and professional.

You're not done. Now, absorb your experience. Grab a piece of paper and ask yourself: What worked? What can you calibrate? What could have worked better? Review any constructive advice that you have received from a director or producer who didn't select you. Focus on improving your areas of weakness. What do you want to concentrate on next time? Now you have clear goals. This is your experience to own.

4. Speech or Presentation

Think in chunks. No matter what the subject, you're telling a story. Remember the order of the story you're about to tell; this way, should you get lost, you'll still know where you are in the story and can easily improvise by continuing with that thread. Should you leave out a line (or fact) or two in the process until you regain your place, only you will know because you are the only one who knew what information you were about to present. Relax.

This is why presentation graphic software programs are so popular. Not only do they provide spiffy visuals to keep your audience engaged, they keep the speaker on-subject and remind them where they are by feeding them speaking points. Magic!

- » Rehearse out loud and get comfortable to your own speaking voice.
- » Learn as much as possible about the setting: lighting, acoustics, temperature, location, and commute time for your performance space.
- » Get yourself in front of a mirror. Try on your chosen clothing, shoes, and hair style before-hand.
- » Be present. Take a few minutes to do deep breathing exercises to loosen up your core. Relax and tell your story.

5. Theater Performance

Again, you're telling a story. Even if you have opening-night jitters, remember the order of the story you're about to tell and that you're not alone. Your fellow actors will be right there with you—trust them. Everyone on that stage has a vested interest in the success of the performance itself. The performance is now an animated, living, breathing creature being born on the spot and everyone has their role. Breathe. Relax. Live the story and the lines will take care of themselves.

Memorization and Preparation

- » **Lines:** Find someone to practice your lines with. Work with different people. You'll quickly find that different things come out of each reading, especially with other actors.
- » **Mix It Up:** Just select arbitrary spots within the piece and finish your lines. Change the tempo of your lines. Change the color of emotion. It's called a play—so play!

» **Evolution Quiz:** You can divide any piece into sections with marks in the margin to identify different phases of the piece with assigned letter names, color codes, or whatever makes you comfortable. Now, can you see how the characters evolve? When fed lines randomly, can you now identify the place in that character's evolution?

Performance preparation includes being able to maintain your focus. Consider running lines while the TV is on some really obnoxious show or have a friend cough, clap, or set off a phone (at random). Even after you've done your dress rehearsal, the actual audience faces and noises can cause you to lose your focus. Most in the audience will not have detected or even minded a blunder. It's a part of live theater. There is absolutely no benefit to worry; focus instead on enjoying playing in this moment. Relax and just tell the story.

The more you work on the numerous skills of your craft, the more you will enjoy exercising those skills.

6. Music Performance

Memorization and preparation again help to steady jangling nerves. So you've memorized key, form, structure, and chord progressions of all the music you're going to perform. Great! Maybe you've also analyzed and executed both note and finger patterns (hands separately). Even better. Now, choose the most difficult sections and repeat this process. Remember, don't just depend on speed and momentum of the particular difficult spot (or the entire piece for that matter) to get you through.

Okay, so now your technique is impeccable. Once you feel that you've got a good technical and musical grasp of the piece, *have some fun with it!*

» **Phrase Quiz:** Divide the piece up into phrases with marks in the margin to identify different phrases in the music with assigned letter names, color codes and so on.

» **Blindfold, Please?:** As you play the piece without the music in front of you see if you can close your eyes and just visualize the exact spots in the music where you're playing.

» **Mix It Up:** Change the tempo from one extreme to another. Transpose a section to a different key completely. Can you sing the left-hand part while the right hand plays alone? Can you sing the next melodic phrase while the left hand plays? Use different dynamics or phrasing.

» **Soloing:** If you've captured the solo of another player or are using rudimentary chord-scales, fire it up by switching colors mid-stream; throw in the unexpected lick and just see where it takes you. They don't call it "playing music" for nothing. Play!

» **Listen to your sound.** You know the music. Remember to listen to the musicians around you. Feel what they're playing—especially the other soloists. Listen! Again, think in chunks or musical phrases. Connect your phrases. Sing your story, and the rest will take care of itself. The music is all there. Trust and let it flow.

All-Purpose Performance Jitter Reduction

Do not spend hours practicing the evening before a performance or the actual day of the performance. The same applies to musicians, dancers, and actors. You've done the work, now trust it.

Focus instead on getting rest and having your mind calmly adjusted to the goal at hand: telling a story while keeping technical aspects under as much control as possible, and keeping focused awareness to what you and the others around you are doing.

Find out the venue and commute time, lighting, acoustics, and temperature of your gig well in advance. Also, check-out your outfit (makeup and hair if needed) the day before so there's no rush on the day of your performance. This way, you keep yourself relaxed and you can anticipate changes. Hydrate well the day before and for up to two hours prior to your actual performance. Some other tips include:

» Do a light warm-up and stretch carefully. Try out specific sections of the pieces but don't over-do it.

» Try to release memories of any mistakes made in rehearsal and be in THIS moment now.

» Anticipate having fun in *this* performance. Smile. See an image of yourself having fun. See in your mind the performance going perfectly and the audience enjoying it!

» BREATHE! Relax.
» Remember the audience is just there to enjoy themselves. They are on your side.
» Feel the tempo in your gut before you start.
» If a memory slip occurs, maintain your posture and rhythm.

Someone asked me, "Aren't stress and anxiety really the same thing?" Nope, although one can cause the other. Anxiety is the actual feeling of nervousness or fear. Stress finds its roots in situations or thoughts that make you feel angry, nervous, worried, frustrated, or even anxious. Things that are stressful to you may not be stressful to someone else.

Being more in terms of life's anxieties begins with recognizing them. Can you now see the need to bring your frustrations forward instead of trying to constantly bury them? Instead, shine a little light in that closet where the monsters are hiding. Maybe you'll gain some understanding. In the midst of the perfect storm, you cannot always just think your way out. There are so many levels of stuff that you're dealing with. But the most important thing you'll achieve is to relieve some of that pressure.

Dance with the elephants!

8

You don't have to sit there for an hour to gain these kinds of benefits. One minute? Three minutes? Ten Minutes? Twenty minutes? Whatcha got?

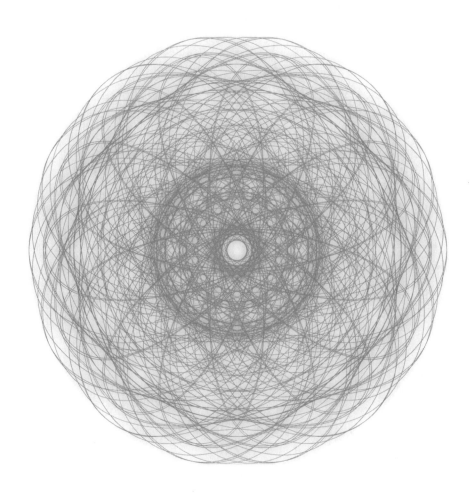

Meditation (Your Mini-Vacation)

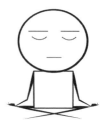

What is meditation? In a nutshell, it can be described as:

» Quieting your mind.
» Releasing yourself from the noise of external and internal distractions.
» Bringing your singular focus to experience quiet and peace.

Sound good? You know that you've been meaning to get around to doing this or that for some time now. So, here's your excuse to start.

Let me guess—you don't have time. You're too exhausted by the end of your day or there's not enough time in the morning to do it. I hear you, but this is about reclaiming time for your *self*.

Here's the short list of benefits:

1. Increases blood flow and slows the heart rate.
2. Decreases respiratory rate and improves flow of air to the lungs, resulting in easier breathing.
3. Produces lasting beneficial changes in brain electrical activity.
4. Greater communication between the two brain hemispheres.
5. Reduces emotional distress and anxiety attacks by lowering the levels of blood lactate.
6. Increases serotonin level, and influences mood and behavior.
7. Improves sleep.
8. Enhances the immune system.
9. Reduces free radicals, which leads to less tissue damage.
10. Harmonizes our endocrine system.
11. Reduces activity of viruses.
12. Lowers cholesterol levels and risk of cardiovascular disease.
13. Decreases the aging process.
14. Higher levels of DHEA (dehydroepiandrosterone).
15. Enhances energy, strength, and vigor.
16. Improves learning ability and enhances memory.

17. Increases feelings of vitality and rejuvenation.
18. Helps with focus and concentration.
19. Increases creativity.
20. Improved performance in athletic events.

That's just the short list!

It's a natural fact that sometimes things become so loaded and over-complicated we can't even get started. You don't have to do anything formal in order to meditate. Really! No equipment is necessary and you don't have to sit there for an hour to gain the benefits listed. One minute? Three minutes? Ten minutes? Twenty minutes? Whatcha got?

Whatever you can spare for yourself is fine. It all will be beneficial.

Easy Meditation Technique

A quiet space indoors or out in nature would be nice, but many of us don't have that luxury. That's okay. We're about to find the quiet space within YOU—the "space between thoughts" as they say. Start wherever you are.

Now, find yourself a comfortable seating position, preferably in a chair with a back, with your spine straight and not slouching. If in a chair, have both feet on the ground, shoulder-width apart. Sitting on the floor? Sit in a cross-legged position. Just be comfortable. Let anticipation and expectation go. Relax. This is easy.

» Close your eyes and breathe as naturally as possible. After a few breaths, try breathing more deeply but with your abdomen only (you learned this earlier in the deep breathing exercise). Feel your stomach rise and the slight movement in the ribcage, collarbones, and shoulders as the breath moves upward. Slowly, your breath will naturally deepen as you do this more often. Focus on the sensation of the movement of air in and out of your nostrils. Try inhaling to a count of 5 and exhaling for the same amount of time.

» Begin to quiet your mind. Of course, any sounds around you will be elevated—just hear them and let them go. Thoughts will come—don't struggle against them. Keep relaxing and consistently bring your consciousness back to your breath. This becomes easier the more you do it.

»   If you have trouble letting go, focus on just one thing, such as a word or mantra that can invoke a calming effect within you, for instance, *Aum*, *Om*, or *I am*. Or imagine an globe of brilliant, diamond-like white light just a foot above your head and feel it radiating down through every aspect of your being and surrounding you with healing and peace. Some find focusing on a sense of gratitude brings feelings of amazing contentment and Joy.

»   Fill your heart with loving warmth and simply sit with that feeling as it radiates through and around you.

»   Even take this time to imagine that perfect beach moment. Feel each sensation of your experience (the sun, smell of the water, a slight cooling breeze, the sound of the waves gently lapping).

Really, really *Be* there. You can use any image you like: splash through Buckingham Fountain in Chicago (feel the silliness) or fly like a condor over the Grand Canyon (feel the freedom); blaze up the Pacific Coast Highway or Route 66 with the top down (feel the exhilaration); imagine money just pouring into your bank account and feel the delight of this wealth; visit with a departed loved one and really feel pleasure in their presence; enjoy a long missed game of tag with a childhood friend. *Laugh!* There are no rules!

This is your time for yourself, your moment. No one need know where you go or what you do. The only two rules are that you feel each sensation of your experience and you enjoy the heck out of it and/or find a sense of astonishing peace.

This is such an instant way to slow down your life for just a few minutes and bring back a little sanity. This really is the very definition of Being more. If I've made it sound incredibly easy do to, that's because it is. You'll find that once you take that giant leap of committing time to yourself, the rest is simple.

In this state of meditation, you are completely in the present moment and only the moment. We all seek clarity. What better way than to turn down the volume of thoughts, worries, concerns, hopes, and prospects so that you can actually think?

Do this for yourself in pockets of time, as much as you feel comfortable with, as often as you can. Hopefully, twice a day you'll find the time to meditate or have a mini-vacation.

9

When a certain brainwave state is experienced and practiced throughout a period of time, the brain will "learn" the state change and it will become easier to self-produce the desired brainwave state at will. The same applies to relaxation.

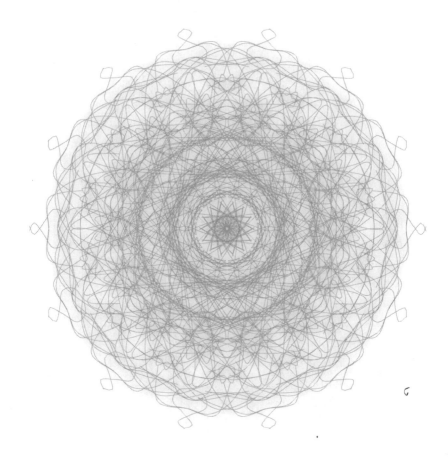

Brainwave Entrainment

This can serve as another tool in your box to clear unhealthy stress. How does it work? Your brain is always active and is comprised of billions of cells called *neurons*, which use electricity to communicate with each other via signals that produce an enormous amount of electrical activity. This clamor can actually be detected using sensitive medical equipment (such as an EEG), measuring electricity levels over areas of your scalp.

When you're alert and focused, you're in what's called the Beta state. Watching television can "zone you out" and move you into a mixture of Beta and the activity level just below it called *Alpha*. In this state, you're generally relaxed or reflective. Theta is an early stage of sleep that is followed by the Delta wave pattern, which is deep sleep. By far these last two are the most interesting brainwave states.

- » Beta (13–40 Hz) Active, alert, and focused.
- » Alpha (8–12 Hz) Relaxed, calm, and creative.
- » Theta (4–8 Hz) Drowsy, light sleep, and dreams.
- » Delta (less than 4 Hz) Deep sleep.

How do they measure all of this? When monitored by an EEG, each type of brain wave signifies a different speed of oscillating electrical voltages in your brain.

As you'll note above, Delta waves are the slowest (zero to four cycles per second) and is present in deep sleep. Theta (four to seven cycles per second) is present in stage one of your sleep cycle when you're in light sleep. Alpha waves, operating at 8 to 13 cycles per second, occur during REM sleep (in addition to when you are awake). Meanwhile, Beta waves, which represent your fastest cycles at 13 to 40 per second, are usually only seen when you're under major stress, including those situations that require very strong mental concentration and focus.

Gamma waves measure somewhere between 25 to 100 cycles (although 40 is most common). Considered by some to be your brain's optimal frequency, Gamma waves are linked with increased compassion, peak brain function, awareness of reality, and increased mental abilities. Reportedly, research with Tibetan Buddhist monks has shown a direct correlation between transcendental mental states and these Gamma waves. Even though they're more rapid than Beta waves, these Gamma brainwaves have almost no noticeable amplitude and can be found in every part of your brain. Gamma waves are believed to improve brain function and perception because they serve as a binding mechanism between all parts of your brain. Let's look a little deeper into the relaxed states, because these are the ones that you most need to access to reduce your stress.

Theta Brain Waves: When they show up on a person's EEG, they will indicate not just early stages of sleep and deep relaxation, but also the process of dreaming. They're high amplitude, and they typically arise when you experience powerful floods of emotion (even those during your dreams). Theta waves have also been identified as a way to access learning and enhanced memory. Yep, this is when sleep learning programs will have their affect by re-activating information recently acquired. Theta meditation reportedly increases creativity, enhances learning (so-called "super learning"), reduces stress, and awakens intuition. Theta waves have been linked to having a strong intuition. This is due to the stronger connection to your unconscious mind or unconscious processing, which heightens advanced problem-solving and learning ability. Some have reported boosted immune system functioning as well.

Delta Brain Waves: This is an indication of your deep stages of sleep (stage 3 and stage 4) and are linked with being completely unconscious (you usually won't know or remember anything while Delta waves are dominant). Your brain lights up when you're in Delta. These waves have been known to oscillate throughout all areas of your brain, and unlike Alpha and Beta, they're usually not synchronized. Of all brainwave ranges, your Delta waves have the greatest amplitude and they surge during demanding mental activities that require concentration.

This is the strongest area of impact for your stress levels because Delta brainwaves have been known to reduce levels of cortisol in your body. Cortisol, as we discussed earlier, is a hormone released when you're under stress that can cause major damage to your body and ultimately destroys brain cells as well. Cortisol has been linked to rapid aging. On the flip side, having less cortisol has been associated with anti-aging. For some people with high amounts of stress, Delta brain waves seem to reduce their adrenaline levels.

Other documented effects of Delta brain waves include the release of human growth hormone (HGH) and melatonin, and some report deeper connection with their intuition. In fact, through meditation, some people can actually learn to increase their Delta activity.

Why is all of this relevant? What if there was some way to simply take your brain from one state to another—to sort of skip ahead or backward in your quest for relaxation?

Through years of study and research, it was discovered that specific sounds could be combined and sequenced to gradually lead our brains through the various states ranging from deep relaxation or sleep, to expanded states of awareness and other "extraordinary" states. *How?*

It's simple, really. Imagine that you have two tuning forks standing side-by-side. When one is struck (causing it to oscillate and resonate) the second tuning fork will automatically begin to oscillate. The first tuning fork is said to have "entrained" the second one or have caused it to resonate.

This same concept applies when a specific brainwave state is experienced and practiced for some period of time, the brain will "learn" the state change. It will also become easier to self-produce the desired brainwave state at will.

So through use of an external stimulus applied to the brain, it is possible to entrain the brainwave frequency to move from one wave state to another. For instance, let's say a person is in the Alpha state (highly alert) and a stimulus of 10Hz is applied to his/her brain for some time. Naturally, the brain frequency will make a gradual shift toward the applied stimulus. The person will experience a gradual relaxation. This phenomenon is the "frequency following response." Research has shown that by using brainwave entrainment, you can expect to get some of its effects later, even without any external stimulus.

But how the heck do we "apply the stimuli?" Well, the easiest, most non-invasive way is via ears and eyes. Because your very human ear cannot hear sounds low enough to be useful for brain stimulation, special techniques must be used. One such special technique used is called "binaural beats."

Binaural literally means "having or relating to two ears." The sensation of "auditory" binaural beats used in brainwave entrainment occur when two clear sounds (of nearly identical frequencies) are presented (one to each ear), through stereo headphones or speakers. Your brain then naturally integrates those two signals, which then produces the sensation of a third sound called the *binaural beat*.

Binaural beats actually originate in your own brain stem's superior olivary nucleus, which is the site of contra-lateral integration of auditory input. So in a nutshell, you've got a different signal being broadcast to each ear, which then creates a third signal that you *experience* in the center as just one sound.

What Is the Relaxation Response?

As mentioned earlier, your brain enters into a few different states throughout the day and night. Each of these states generates its own measureable and unique frequency. Brainwave entrainment, by broadcasting waves specifically in the delta and theta level range, will ease your brain waves directly into a natural relaxation response. This mental, physical, and emotional state is characterized by lowered blood pressure, decreased heart, breathing, "metabolic rates," and mind/body coherence—all good things.

Harvard professor Dr. Herbert Benson, founder of the Mind/Body Medical Institute at Boston's Deaconess Hospital, coined the term "relaxation response."[1] Through research, he concluded that this relaxation response produces many long-term health benefits (in addition to the immediate effects created during the brainwave entrainment experience). This is an effective method to trigger the natural healing mechanisms of your body!

Physically, the relaxation response will:

» Decrease blood pressure and slow heart rate.
» Diminish respiration rate and reduce oxygen consumption (hypometabolism).
» Relax muscles.

Mental benefits include:

» Clears the mind from anxiety.
» Creates a feeling of calm and peacefulness.
» Changes brainwave frequencies (generally slowing from Beta to Theta/Delta).

Is this cheating? Well, sort of. We're so often challenged for time—a little nudge that is non-drug-related seems acceptable. Brainwave entrainment use can bring not only deep relaxation, but also enhanced meditation, insomnia reduction, and symptoms of stress.

Theta Waves for Enhanced Learning— a Deeper Look

Research has found that during your dream sleep (REM sleep), meditation, peak experiences, and creative states, your brain is in Theta brainwave territory. REM sleep (Theta brainwaves) is a big part of the process by which creativity blends associative elements into brand new combinations that are useful to you. In other words, when your brain is producing Theta waves, the unconscious or suppressed parts of your psyche, as well as your creativity are boosted, which is why it's said to inspire insight or creative leaps. *How?*

Biology 101: There are two parts of your brain that are important: the hippocampus (that's the big frontal lobe of your brain where you do all of your consolidation of information from short-term memory to long-term memory and your spatial navigation from point A to point B) and neo-cortex (where all of your motor commands, spatial reasoning, conscious thought, and language happen).

When your brain is producing those Theta waves, high levels of acetylcholine in your hippocampus suppress information moving to your neo-cortex. Now, those lower levels of acetylcholine and norepinephrine in your neo-cortex will boost the spread of associational activity within your entire neocortical areas without control coming in from your pesky hippocampus. This is the complete opposite of what happens in your consciousness when you're wide-awake, where increased levels of norepinephrine and acetylcholine actually *hold back* repeated connections with your neo-cortex.

As long as you only produce Theta brainwaves, their content will remain difficult to get to for your waking (conscious) mind. You need Alpha waves to bridge that gap between Theta and Beta brainwaves in order to consciously experience or remember content from the Theta state.

A Weizmann Institute study appearing in the August 2012 *Nature Neuroscience* clearly showed that learned responses are more prominent during your REM sleep (Theta brainwave) phase, but the *transfer* of the associations from sleep to waking could be proven only when learning took place during the non-REM phase. Study researchers Anat Arzi and Noam Sobel suggest that during REM sleep, you may be more open to influence from information (or stimuli) in your surroundings, but so-called "dream amnesia"—which makes you forget most of your dreams—may also operate on any conditioning which happens in that stage of sleep. So the stand-out difference is the non-REM sleep is the phase that is important for your memory consolidation, which means it might also play an important role in your ability to "sleep-learn."[2]

So, to say you "learn" during REM sleep or Theta brainwave activity is not as really as accurate as to say that information you have absorbed consciously (wide-awake) is actually deeply imprinted or absorbed during your sleep or Theta brainwave activity. Brainwave entrainment has been used to generate this Theta wave state.

Much research has been done to advance the usage of brainwave entrainment, and in the back of this book you'll find information on where you can pick up CDs or download tracks that employ them for use in relaxation, meditation, and improved focus for studying.

It's another tool for you to consider in slowing down the flurry of life so that you can Be more.

10

This is how you assimilate emotional and mental events of your previous day and reset your mind for the day ahead.

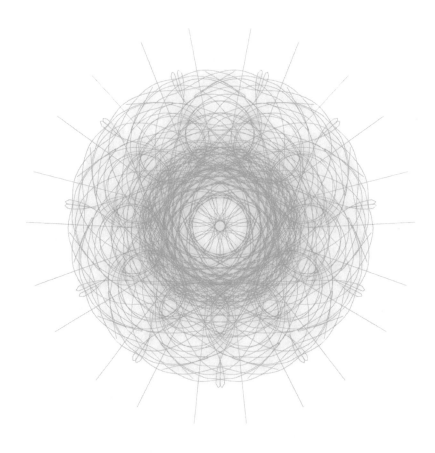

Sleep (Get More!)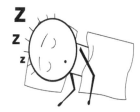

So, you're all ready to go nighty-night and you expect your brain and body to switch off as easily as you switch off the lights. Yet for many people, that's simply not possible. We either can't fall asleep easily or stay asleep peacefully. What's going on? Let's take a deeper look.

Let's peek into the effects of all that sleep you are missing. This is for extensive purposes only! Don't worry, we're going to get into some solutions too.

A 2014 University of Texas Health Science Center study found that people with insomnia are 10 times more likely to be depressed and anxious.[1] Does this surprise you? Beyond the emotional effects, there's the mental effects from lack of sleep as well. "Your ability to learn tasks, and retain and process memory are boosted during sleep," says James Wyatt, PhD, director of the Sleep Disorders Service and Research Center at Rush University Medical Center in Chicago.[2] "The immediate risk of a bad night's sleep is a heightened risk of auto or work accidents," says Dr. Gary Richardson, senior researcher at Henry Ford Sleep Disorders and Research Center in Detroit. "When you have had relatively little sleep—like 4 hours of sleep instead of 8—you can no longer do more than one task at a time," says Richardson.[3] You probably don't think of it this way because it's become second nature, but while driving you are multi-tasking as your brain monitors not only your car's speed, but also the cars around you and road conditions too.

Of course, there're the negative effects of missed sleep on your physical health as well. A 2013 Swedish study proved that just missing a single night of sleep may cause a loss in brain tissue. "We observed that a night of total sleep loss was followed by increased blood concentrations of NSE and S-100B. These brain molecules typically rise in blood under conditions of brain damage. Thus, our results indicate that a lack of sleep may promote neurodegenerative processes," says sleep researcher Christian Benedict at the Department of Neuroscience, Uppsala University, and leader of the study.[4]

There was also a large 5-year study done in 2007 at Warwick Medical School in Coventry, England, that found women who consistently got 6 hours of sleep per night were 42 percent more likely to develop high blood pressure than those who got the standard 7 to 8 hours of nightly shut-eye.[5]

Also, when you're sick, your immune system naturally increases your need for sleep to help it battle and recover from infection, Wyatt says.[6] So "when you're sleep-deprived, your immune system doesn't have the resources it needs to fully fight off infections," leaving you vulnerable to illness, he says.[7] A 2003 study at the Université Laval in Canada confirms this. Researchers there tested blood samples of insomniacs, and found fewer infection-fighting cells than in people who get more sleep.[8]

So your immune system, already compromised by your stress level, takes a hard hit from lack of sleep as well. Researchers from the University of Helsinki have now proven what kinds of biological mechanisms related to sleep loss affect your immune system and trigger a very dangerous inflammatory response.[9] "We compared the gene expression before and after the sleep deprivation period, and focused on the genes whose behavior was most strongly altered," explained lead researcher Vilma Aho.[10] "The expression of many genes and gene pathways related to the functions of the immune system was increased during the sleep deprivation. There was an increase in activity of B cells, which are responsible for producing antigens that contribute to the body's defensive reactions, but also to allergic reactions and asthma. This may explain the previous observations of increased asthmatic symptoms in a state of sleep deprivation."[11] The same research group also found that inflammation increased. "On the gene level, this was apparent in the higher-than-normal expression of the TLR4 gene after sleep loss,"[12] reported the University of Helsinki researchers. "C Reactive Protein level was also elevated, indicating inflammation."[13]

So the bottom line here is, sleep not only impacts your brain function, but also interacts with your immune system and metabolism. "Sleep loss causes changes to the system that regulates our immune defense. Some of these changes appear to be long-term, and may contribute to the development of diseases that have been linked to sleep deprivation in epidemiological research," Aho stated.[14]

But you are far from alone. Sleep deprivation is so commonplace these days that you might not even realize you suffer from it. Are you getting consistently "good" sleep? *Eight full uninterrupted hours?*

Circadian? It's a Rhythm, but Can You Dance to It?

Everything in nature has a rhythm, and that includes your body. The rising and setting of the sun, the ebb and flow of the ocean's tide, and the transition from one season to another all happen with comforting regularity. Circadian rhythms are quite simply the 24-hour biological cycles that maintain time for your body. They're involved in body temperature, hormone secretion, mood disorders, sleep, metabolism, weight gain, heart activity, blood pressure, oxygen consumption, and a variety of diseases.

All of you biological rhythms are based on the 24-hour cycle of daylight and darkness, as well as the monthly cycles of the moon. Just like the monthly biological clock in females, both men and women have 24-hour daily clocks. This is why most of us naturally feel like waking when the sun comes up and sleeping when it's dark. Throughout your day at different times, so-called "clock genes" will signal your body when to produce specific proteins, and the level of these proteins will rise and fall in rhythmic patterns. "These oscillating biochemical signals control various functions, including when we sleep and rest, and when we are awake and active," says the Genetics Science Learning Lab of the University of Utah."[15]

But your internal clock does much more than just help you fall asleep at night. We're all aware that changes in female hormone production vary with a monthly cycle, but cortisol (the adrenal hormone most involved with stress) varies in everyone through a 24-hour or circadian cycle. Your cortisol levels will peak in the early morning hours as the sun rises and taper off as the sun sets. It reaches its lowest levels three hours after dark. This daily rhythm of cortisol dictates when you should be at your most active and when you should rest. Even a time change of just a few hours can be enough to throw off your normal sleep cycle. Why does this matter? Cortisol not only dictates your sleep and wake states, it's also the primary hormone involved in leading your proper immune system function.

As your cortisol levels drop during the evening, your immune cells become more active. Good stuff! While you are at rest, these cells leave the bone marrow and spleen to protect you.

You've probably heard time and time again that without sufficient sleep, your immune system is weakened and therefore challenged to keep up with its repair work. During this highly active period of immune function, your immune cells eliminate cancer cells, bacteria, viruses, and other harmful agents. Essential to this immune activity is that your body has correct levels of cortisol. As your body continues its circadian rhythm dance, at daylight your cortisol level rises and your immune cells return to the bone marrow and spleen to rest and retune in preparation for your next nightly cycle.

Your immune system functions optimally if you to go to sleep by 10 p.m. (oh, did I just lose you?) As you sleep, vital physical repair takes place in addition to the extremely important immune system activities we just discussed. However, if your cortisol remains elevated at night, necessary physical repair work and this crucial immune function is compromised. This creates the opportunity for disease processes to begin.

How about this aspect? As you sleep, you are going into rapid eye movement (or REM) sleep states and non-REM sleep, alternating between light sleep and deep dream states—"maintenance time"—but this is for that amazing brain of yours. This is how you assimilate emotional and mental events of your previous day and reset your mind for the day ahead. Most people need seven to eight hours of sleep to accomplish all of this. So, if you're missing proper rest, both your physical repair and mental regeneration are impaired. *Not good!*

Waking Before the Alarm Clock? It's Just Stress...

Remember that cortisol is naturally at a higher level in the morning than at any other time in your day.

Let's take a look at some research from the University Lübeck in Germany. Their study determined that, for some, anticipating the time you want to get up seems to trigger the release of the exact same neuro-hormones normally secreted by your body in times of stress. Both adrenocorti-cotropin (or ACTH, a hormone produced and secreted by your pituitary gland) and our good friend cortisol are released by your body in anticipation of a stressful event (a big meeting, an exam, an interview, a lion chasing you, and so on). It seems that roughly an hour before you've actually planned to wake up, these secretions increase in preparation for the "stress" of waking.[16] This can't just be a coincidence. Although generally science considers sleep as a state of unconsciousness, clearly the study's findings show your mind may actually have some sort of conscious, voluntary control.

How'd they determine that? At midnight for three consecutive nights, Jan Born and his team tucked 15 sleepy volunteers into bed. They were told that they would be awakened at 6 a.m. their first night and at 9 a.m. the next two nights. That first night, when the volunteers knew that they would be awakened at 6 a.m., their levels of the central stress neuro-hormone ACTH began rising at around 4:30 a.m. Here's where it got interesting. On the next two nights, when they expected to wake at 9 a.m., they were instead rudely awakened at 6 a.m.; the volunteers experienced no hormonal surge *at all*. Conclusion: Your unconscious mind actually notes the time that you anticipate waking and gradually prepares your brain for consciousness by increasing your levels of stress hormones.

Theoretically, awakening in a heightened state of stress may have served early Homo sapiens quite well. Knowing, as we do, that they were not treated to nightly stays at the local Motel 7, one can imagine that there was a need to have the ability to immediately respond to a predator lurking nearby upon waking. Sleep was a dangerous and potentially deadly necessity.

On a small scale, this stress hormone surge has the potential to explain why many report having more active or bad dreams before waking—a time that coincides with their unconscious mind interpreting this new chemical information it's receiving. However, this rise in stress hormones is possibly one of the reasons for the disproportionately high rate of morning heart attacks, which also, as it turns out, are more severe. Heart attacks are five to six times more likely to occur in the early morning hours between 1 and 5 a.m.

Cardiologists have known for some time about this type of heart attack, called ventricular fibrillation, which most often occurs in the morning and is caused by a rapid irregular heartbeat. The heart simply cannot pump blood efficiently as it loses the regularity of beat. In fact, levels of a protein called KLF15 (kruppel-like factor 15) fluctuate while following that circadian clock of yours that we just discussed, which governs the hormonal rhythms throughout your body. Researchers at Baylor College of Medicine report that having too low or too high levels of KLF15 begins a domino effect of events that change the potassium current, which in turn negatively affect the electrical recovery time of your heart muscle cells, so KLF15 becomes a definite factor.[17]

Make-Up Sleep

Really? You thought you could go without sleep and then store it up like a squirrel stores nuts for the winter?

A typical scenario: You're constantly sleep deprived during weekdays and try to catch up on the weekend. Although you might even feel that you've recovered after this extended sleep treat, research shows that the next time you try to go without shut-eye, your performance starts to deteriorate *and* you put yourself at risk for serious metabolic dysfunction, cardiovascular disease, insulin resistance, and obesity.

Research by psychiatrist William C. Dement, founder of the Stanford University Sleep Clinic, suggests that we may accumulate sleep debt surreptitiously. His work shows that even your short-term sleep deprivation can lead to "brain fog," memory loss, worsened vision, and impaired mechanical skills (including driving).[18]

In a study conducted by Fred W. Turek, professor of neurobiology and physiology and director of Northwestern's Center for Sleep and Circadian Biology, chronic (or continual) partial sleep loss of even two to three hours per night was found to have detrimental effects on the body, leading to impairments in cardiovascular, immune, and endocrine functions, as well as cognitive performance; we're talking about everything from depression to high blood pressure.[19] Performance on tasks declined in sleep-restricted people even while they reported not feeling sleepy. These findings support what other research has exposed in recent studies.

Allostatic (a fancy word for "short-term") responses are adaptive—your body will snap back. So, for instance, people who lose sleep because of a single all-nighter can make up for it by boosting the amount of deep sleep they get the next night, says study coauthor Aaron Laposky, also from Northwestern.[20] Deep sleep restores your alertness and helps to keep your memory and other brain functions at optimal levels. On the flipside, studies show that after 24 hours without sleep, your performance can drop to the level equal to that of someone who is legally drunk. So, when sleep deprivation is sustained on a continual basis, such as the volunteers in their study, an allostatic load will develop and actually lead to very serious health outcomes. Making matters even worse, the allostatic load that results from your mounting sleep debt loops back to your natural sleep regulatory system itself and alters that as well.

"Even though animals and humans may be able to adapt their sleep system to deal with repeated sleep restriction conditions, there could be negative consequences when this pattern is maintained over a long period of time," said Turek.[21]

Sunlight also makes a difference in all of this. Sleep debt has been found to be most noticeable during your nighttime activities. Why?

Because research show that your natural tendency for wakefulness during the day may cover up signs of sleep debt when it's light out, but this protective effect may easily disappear as the darkness of night sets in.

Of course, the findings are particularly important for people who work odd-hour jobs, which require going without sleep for extended periods, such as nurses, health workers, truckers, cabbies, and emergency responders. Ironically, these are people who we rely on to be alert, react quickly, and make excellent decisions. This means that among the potentially covert consequences, chronic sleep loss could possibly leave people more vulnerable to accidents and errors, according to research by Daniel Cohen of Brigham and Women's Hospital in Boston, Mass.[22]

What can you do? If you have been chronically sleep deprived, take it easy for a few months (yes, months) to get back into a natural sleep pattern, says Lawrence J. Epstein, medical director of the Harvard-affiliated Sleep Health Centers. In order to get your recovery sleep, both the number of hours slept and the intensity of the sleep are key.[23]

Actually go to bed when you are tired (what a concept), then allow your body to wake naturally (on its own, no alarm clock allowed) in the morning. Initially, your recovery sleep pattern may leave you feeling slightly "catatonic," but don't panic. In fact, expect to store more than 10 hours shut-eye per night. You'll experience a natural and gradual decrease in your amount of sleep time.

Trouble in Paradise

It's possible that what your relationship really needs is just a good night's sleep...in separate beds. Yep, I said it. Dr. Robert Meadows, a sociologist at the University of Surrey, conducted research that shows that people actually feel that they sleep better when they are with a partner, but that's not true.[24] To compare how well couples slept when they shared a bed, contrasted with sleeping separately, Dr. Meadows conducted a very simple study. Using 40 volunteer couples, it revealed that there's a 50 percent chance that a slumbering partner will be disturbed when the couples share a bed and one of them moves in his or her sleep. There's nothing quite like the resentment build-up you experience while watching your partner snoring away blissfully as you are wide awake beside them.

Earlier, pop culture strongly implied that sleeping in separate beds was a sign of "trouble in paradise" hurtling toward the atomic mushroom cloud of marital doom. However, it seems more and more couples are re-thinking that concept in favor of a good night's sleep. According to the U.S. National Sleep Foundation (yes, we have one), couples sleeping separately nearly doubled from 12 percent in 2001 to 23 percent in 2005.[25] According to the National Association of Home Builders, there has been a consistent escalation in requests for "two master bedroom" homes. They go further to predict that by 2015, 60 percent of all custom upscale homes will be built with two "owner suites."[26] Separate beds—food for thought. Speaking of which…

Is Your Body Clock Making You Fat?

The evidence confirms that losing sleep has been shown to have a harmful impact on your fat cells, reducing their ability to respond to insulin (a hormone that regulates your energy) by as much as 30 percent, a process that can lead to weight gain, Type-2 diabetes, and other health problems.

But we're ahead of ourselves—first there's the craving factor. Unfortunately, when we're sleep-deprived, it has been proven that we eat more sugary, salty, high-carb foods such as pancakes and sweet-rolls, says Dr. Gary Richardson, a senior researcher at Henry Ford Sleep Disorders and Research Center in Detroit.[27]

Then it gets more serious. "Not getting enough sleep impairs metabolic processes, disrupting the regulation of glucose levels," says Dr. Wyatt.[28] It was only recently, in 1999, that this connection was made through a University of Chicago study. The researchers used two groups: half of the 27 healthy adults were allowed less than 6½ hours of sleep for 8 days, while the other half had the standard 7½ to 8½ hours of shut-eye. Blood tests revealed that the deprived half produced, on average,

50 percent more insulin and their sensitivity to the hormone was 40 percent lower than the group allowed to sleep the standard amount of time. "The sleep-deprived (group results) looked like they were pre-diabetic," says Dr. Richardson.[29]

But *why* does this happen? "We found that fat cells need sleep to function properly," said Matthew Brady, PhD, associate professor of medicine and vice-chair of the Committee on Molecular Metabolism and Nutrition at the University of Chicago.[30]

According to Brady, body fat plays a vital role in humans. "Many people think of fat as a problem, but it serves a vital function," he said. "Body fat, also known as adipose tissue, stores and releases energy. In storage mode, fat cells remove fatty acids and lipids from the circulation where they can damage other tissues. When fat cells cannot respond effectively to insulin, these lipids leach out into the circulation, leading to serious complications."[31]

During a University of Chicago study, after four nights of short sleep (4½ hours), participants' total-body insulin response was reduced by an average of 16 percent. Also, the insulin sensitivity of their fat cells decreased by 30 percent. Again, the significance of those numbers is comparable to the difference between cells from people with diabetes versus those who are non-diabetic. Do these results motivate you?

But the results went even further. They found that the sleep-deprived study participants had a decreased response to a range of doses of insulin. An increase of nearly three times as much insulin was required to provoke just half of the maximum "Akt response" in volunteers who had been deprived of sleep. *What's Akt?* It's a special kind of enzyme that modifies proteins and plays a key role in multiple cellular processes in your body, such as your glucose metabolism (use of sugars) and the way your cells thrive, die off, or even migrate.

Witnessing the direct effect of sleep deprivation on a peripheral tissue, such as fat, at the cellular level "was an eye-opener," said Josiane Broussard, PhD, lead author of the study. This helps reinforce the link between sleep and diabetes and "suggests that we could use sleep, like diet and exercise to prevent or treat this common disease."[32]

Yet another aspect of sleep loss that directly affects your weight gain is the increase it causes in two hormones linked with your appetite and eating behavior. More specifically, lack of sleep reduces leptin (a hormone that tells your brain that there is no need for more food) and increases ghrelin (a hormone that triggers hunger). *Translation?* You're hungrier and it becomes difficult to even recognize when you're full.

On the other hand, your diet also impacts your internal clock, because what you eat sends your body signals about when to wake up and go to sleep. This means that spacing your meals at relatively consistent times throughout the day will help to reinforce other time-setting activities.

This is one reason why it's best not to eat a big meal right before you go to bed; this tells your body to get to work digesting your food during a time when it should be signaling you to go to sleep. Try not to eat or drink within two hours of your bedtime. However, maintaining optimum blood sugar levels is always the most important consideration for your health. So if you are hungry at a late hour, then having a small 200-calorie snack, preferably one that includes protein, is fine (like a handful of raw walnuts). Just don't have a massive meal at a late hour. Having a lot of liquid late-night means disrupted sleep for that trip to the bathroom, so try to get your liquids in earlier in the day.

How Does Disrupted Circadian Rhythm Cause Cancer?

Aside from weight gain, if you throw your internal clock off kilter too much, chronic diseases like cancer can result. In fact, the Journal of the National Cancer Institute[33] recently added overnight shift work to the list of probable carcinogens, because it disrupts your circadian rhythm. This disruption may influence cancer progression through shifts in important neuro-hormones like melatonin, secreted by the pineal gland in increased levels toward evening prompting sleep, which is known to suppress tumor development.

Melatonin is an antioxidant that helps to suppress harmful free radicals (cellular byproducts) in your body and slows the production of estrogen, which can activate cancer. When your circadian rhythm is disrupted, your body may produce less melatonin and therefore may have less ability to fight cancer.

A Completely Dark Bedroom Is a Necessity!

So here's the thing. DEEP inside the eye they've discovered these photo-sensitive ganglia. *Huh?!*

Biology 101: Back when we were little one-celled amoeba happily swimming around in the primordial soup, we didn't have eyes. Nope. There was really nothing to see—not even land masses. The one thing we needed to know about for our survival was when it was dark and when it was light, which happily coincided with when it was time to eat or to rest. Hence, photo-sensitive ganglia responsive to light allowed us to know when we could surface safely to feed, or when to submerge. The sun's ultra-violet light would've killed us if we stayed up during full sunlight. So we developed specific sensitivity to yellow light and blue light waves. Blue meant the sun was high; we needed to be alert and cautious. Yellow meant the longer rays of the sun as it lowered were now present—it was safe to feed, and as darkness fell, to rest. Don't worry; this all comes together to make a point in the following paragraph.

If we discount what some argue is mythical evidence that the Egyptians had electric light, thereby explaining the absence of any signs of soot within the elaborately decorated windowless pharaonic tombs, then Humphry Davy, an English chemist, is the culprit who invented the *first* electric light in 1809.[34] Yes, here's that man that enabled us to be up at all hours with our darned convenient street lights, head lights, porch lights, ceiling lights, lamps by the sofa, in the bathroom, in the hallway ("Honey can you turn off that light in the kitchen? You're wasting electricity.") We are *lit* up! Some go so far as to call it light pollution.

All of this artificial lighting is dimmer and less "blue-weighted" than natural daylight, contributing to age-related losses in our unconscious circadian photo-reception. You see, we never lost the original photo-receptive ganglia that we started with—they're still there. They're called intrinsically photosensitive retinal ganglion cells (ipRGC) or melanopsin for short.

Sure, we later developed the familiar rods and cones you learned about in science class that allow us to see images, but all of our convenience lighting has doused our natural sensitivity to the lengthening of the sun's rays—the "dimming of the day." The yellows, oranges, and pinks have lost their effectiveness. We miss our cue to settle down and relax. Now we've compounded this because we stare for hours upon end into gadgets and computer screens that emit tons of blue light. Guess what that does?! It seriously disrupts your body's signal to create melatonin.

Not to beat a "life-challenged" horse, but to give you slightly more detail, there's a part of your brain called the suprachiasmatic nucleus (SCN)—*I know, that's a lot of syllables*—which is a group of cells in your hypothalamus that controls your circadian clock by responding to light and dark signals.

Light actually travels through your eye's optic nerve to your SCN, where it then signals your body's clock that it's time to wake up. Light also signals your SCN to initiate other processes associated with being awake, such as raising your body temperature and producing hormones like cortisol.

On the opposite side, when your eyes signal to your SCN that it's dark outside, your body will begin to produce melatonin. The more your sleep is disrupted by light pollution, the lower your melatonin levels (and the greater your risk of developing cancer becomes).

As mentioned earlier, melatonin, which is secreted predominantly in your brain at night, activates a multitude of biochemical actions, including a nocturnal reduction in your body's estrogen levels. It's thought that chronically decreasing your melatonin production at night, which happens when you're exposed to nighttime light, actually increases your risk of developing cancer.

There was a very important study done linking cancer to light, which showed that blind women have a 36-percent lower risk of breast cancer compared to sighted women. *Why?* Simply because they are unreceptive to light. This means that their bodies maintain high melatonin levels *regardless* of how much light is in the room.

"Basically, what we found is that chronic exposure to bright light—even the kind of light you experience in your own living room at home or in the workplace at night if you are a shift worker—elevates levels of a certain stress hormone in the body, which results in depression and lowers cognitive function," said Samer Hattar, a biology professor in the Johns Hopkins University's Krieger School of Arts and Sciences. He conducted a 2012 study entitled, "Aberrant light directly impairs mood and learning through melanopsin-expressing neurons."[35] "I'm not saying we have to sit in complete darkness at night, but I do recommend that we should switch on fewer lamps, and stick to less-intense light bulbs: basically, only use what you need to see. That won't likely be enough to activate those ipRGCs that affect mood," he advises.[36]

So, whatcha gonna do?!

Mitigation

If you've been on your computer for eight hours, then your brain has been receiving the signal that it is "high noon" for eight hours. Give it a break! Some may experience more agitation from this than others, but all are over-stimulated by the effect.

> » Get blue-blocking eyewear to use at night and while using your computer for lengths of time.
> » Install blackout drapes or shades in your bedroom.
> » Close your bedroom door if light comes through it (even simply put a towel along the base to prevent light from seeping in).
> » Remove your electric clock radio (or at least cover it up at night and be sure to get one that has red numbers).
> » Avoid night lights or consider getting the special yellow-orange kind.

This all probably sounds pretty extreme. It's difficult to fully appreciate the power of this simple yet effective intervention. However, most people are shocked at how much better they feel when they improve the quality of their sleep.

So You're a Night Owl; What Should You Do?

What if you're a "night person" and simply feel best working and staying awake at night and sleeping during the day? It's important to ask whether you truly feel better this way or if it is more a matter of habit, convenience, or other exterior reason why you've adjusted your schedule this way.

Consider for a moment that people have naturally been sleeping during the nighttime for many millenia, before the arrival of electricity and the Internet.

If your life circumstances lead you to the conclusion that staying up at night is non-negotiable—for instance if you consistently work the night shift and can't change it—you can somewhat counter the health effects by still maintaining a specific schedule. This way, your body's clock will eventually adjust to your personal sleep/wake cycle and this is less damaging than if you constantly change shifts and expect your body clock to follow along with you. People who frequently have insomnia, travel long distances, or must change from day shifts to night shifts often, find themselves in this situation.

The bottom line here is that your body is an extraordinary source of feedback. The key is to honor the signals your body is giving you.

Pests That Go Bump in the Night

Oh yeah…we all get 'em. One minute you're asleep, the next you're wide awake with your thoughts running wild. *STRESS!* Or worse, you can't get to sleep at all. I've got a couple of amazingly simple techniques to silence the pests!

Mitigation

» **Attention List**: Before you go to bed, write down any lingering thoughts ("to-do" lists, conversations left incomplete or which need to be had, memories that loop). Place them all into list form on a sheet of paper with the intent and knowledge that they will be addressed the following day, but for now must be put away to allow your mind and body the precious time it needs to relax and re-vitalize. This simple tool puts your unconscious mind more at ease, because you now have consciously acknowledged those lose threads.

Be certain to list a few of the things that you accomplished that are positive during your day. It's important to also recognize achievements, and we sometimes forget to give ourselves a much-needed pat on the back.

You'll be amazed at how this simple little tool can transform your life. When you review these lists from time to time, you'll begin to notice patterns that creep-up in your life—repeated issues that you can now see clearly need some attention—*just not when you're about to go to bed!*

» **Liberation Word**: So you're lying there, things going back and forth in your mind. You check the clock counting down to wake-up time. The thoughts keep coming. Believe it or not this is a remnant of your speech center development, which starts at about 3 months old. You've seen babies randomly cooing, gurgling, and making otherwise unintelligible sounds, which their parents will swear that they understand. Your speech center "practices" sounds repetitively as you develop language skills. But in this instance your subconscious anxieties and stress have co-opted this little tool. Well, here's a great trick to reclaim your head space.

As soon as you realize that you're thought rambling—and sometimes it may take a while to even recognize this—use the liberation word that you've selected. (Mine is *zucchini* for no particular reason other than I like the sound of it.) Begin repeating your liberation word quietly in your head. Free your mind! It will gradually displace or crowd-out your rambling thoughts and you'll begin to drift back to sleep.

In a similar way to the brainwave entrainment discussed previously, as you use this tool more and more, less repetitions of your liberation word will be necessary to carry you back into peaceful slumber.

Sleep Hygiene

We must take a little "holiday" in the two hours before bed. *You must train yourself to relax* even if you have to patiently coerce the sensation by lying in the dark and consciously, gently relaxing each body part and emptying your mind—*several times*—to truly unwind. Use these simple tips to get between seven and nine hours of sleep, which as we've just learned, can have dramatic positive effects on your weight and health:

- » Avoid substances known to affect sleep, such as sugar, caffeine, and alcohol.
- » Avoid any stimulating activities for two hours before bed, such as using the Internet, texting, answering e-mails, or watching TV.
- » Put on eyewear to block out blue light two to three hours prior to bedtime (even better right after sunset).
- » Don't eat or drink within 2 hours of bedtime.
- » Create a sleep ritual. It sounds corny, but have a special set of little things that you consistently do before bed to help ready your system physically and psychologically for sleep. This can guide your body into a deep, healing sleep.
- » Try to get daily exposure to daylight for at least 20 minutes. That sunlight enters your eyes and triggers the release of specific brain chemicals and hormones (like melatonin) that are vital to healthy sleep, mood, and aging.
- » Exercise daily for 20 minutes (but not three hours before bed, which can affect sleep).

» Keep a routine sleep schedule. Go to bed and wake at the same time each day.

» Make an appealing environment for yourself that encourages sleep by eliminating clutter and using peaceful, restful colors.

» Use your bed only for sleep and sexual activities.

» Keep your bedroom very dark or use eyeshades.

» Block out sound if you have a noisy environment by using earplugs (soft silicone ones work well) or a white noise machine.

» Make the room a comfortable temperature for sleep.

» Write out your Attention List.

» Do deep breathing exercises for at least 5 to 15 minutes just before you get into bed.

» Get a massage or do some gentle stretching.

» Have a warm salt/soda aromatherapy bath. Raising your body temperature before bed helps to induce sleep. A warm bath also relaxes your muscles and reduces tension physically and psychologically. By adding half a cup to 1 cup of epsom salt (magnesium sulfate) and ½ to 1 cup of baking soda (sodium bicarbonate) to your bath, you will gain the benefits of magnesium absorbed through your skin and the alkaline-balancing effects of the baking soda, both of which aid sleep. You might even add 10 drops of lavender essential oil to your bathwater.

Some Nutritional Supplementation to Consider for Sleep

» Consider relaxing minerals such as magnesium citrate or glycinate before bed (which relaxes the nervous system and muscles). It is best to take magnesium with calcium (at a 1:1 ratio 500mgs).

» Herbal remedies may help. Consider passion flower or valerian (valeriana officinalis) root extract (standardized to 0.2 percent valerenic acid), vhamomile, holy basil, kava kava, wild lettuce leaf extract, suma, skullcap, ashwagandha, or lemon balm one hour before bed. Other supplements and herbs can be helpful in getting some shut-eye, such as L-Theanine (an amino acid from green tea), glycine powder, GABA, 5-HTP, and magnolia. You can experiment with herbal combinations or blends to find the best effect for you. Melatonin supplementation is a popular choice.

Among other reasons, know that you deserve a good, peaceful nights' slumber to allow yourself to de-stress, renew, and rejuvenate the mind, body and spirit.

Conclusion

"To be nobody but yourself in a world which is doing its best, night and day, to make you everybody else, means to fight the hardest battle which any human being can fight; and never stop fighting."

—*e.e. cummings*[1]

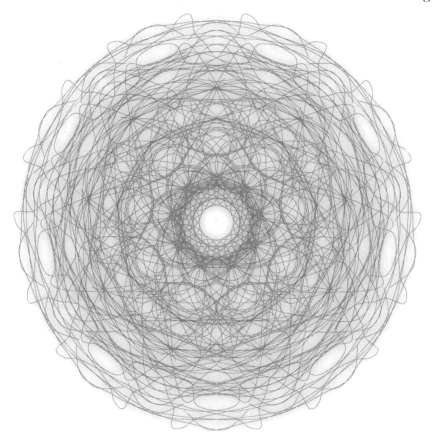

Conclusion

Who are we really? Are we who our peers or parents believe we are? Are we our unconscious? Are we the catalog and summation of our experiences? Are we our ideals, hopes, and dreams? Or are we the interpretation we make and value we assign to all of these? How can we even know or focus while we're in a constant swirl of chaos?

Slow down. Just claim "I'm slowing it all down" and reclaim some time for your self. Stress is no longer an option—it's far too damaging. Remember it is how you perceive your stress that really matters.

Remember the example of the out-of-control car set in a spin? You need to keep your eyes on where you want to be and keep steering toward it. Drop the mask and take care of the inner things that are hurting you. Many develop bad habits and self-sabotaging, self-destructive behaviors because they feel victimized by life and don't feel deserving of love, health, good food, and other ways of nurturing and pleasuring themselves. We've seen how misperceptions accumulate throughout a lifetime and have a domino effect across the full spectrum of health.

Cultivating self-love is a *very* over-simplified concept, but know that you are unique—there's no one exactly like you. The same spark in you that sustains your life is that which sustains the very universe itself and in that you are connected more than you could ever imagine to something grand. If no one has said this to you lately (or ever), you are wonder-full.

Love is your birthright. You are connected to it in the same way that you are connected to the non-local energy of the cosmos, because it is of that same energy, we simply recognize it in different ways and forms.

Here's an easier way to see it. When you slip a teaspoon of sugar into a warm glass of water, it dissolves. In fact, it mixes *so* completely that you cannot remove it again as a simple teaspoon of sugar. Now apply this same simple concept to the original non-local energy that formed everything in your awareness *including* the energy *of* your awareness itself. You see it now. It's all of that single original source (Big Bang)—we simply identify that energy now in altered forms—a chair, a lamp, a dove, a seal, a computer, the sun, the moon, you, me, the deep blue sea. It's still all one energy and you can raise the level of your vibration to match the form we call Love—at your will. It requires only that you remember it—enlivening your *perception* of it. You can use your meditation to strengthen your connection to both Love and Joy. That we are spirits (energy) having a physical experience is never more pertinent than when we're under stress.

Be kind. It costs you nothing and truly you contribute so much to just making this world a gentler and less stressful place. Take a moment to look into the eyes of each person you are speaking with. The point is that from CEO, to check-out clerk, to custodial engineer, there is a human commonality that we should recognize in one another. Being indifferent, speaking thoughtlessly, acting selfishly—in these moments, ask yourself What do I really gain through this behavior? Is this the world that I want to create? Don't hoard your Joy—share it.

Whether you feel it or not, you are powerful. You get to create and recreate your life in each moment by the thoughts that you choose. Redirect your thoughts the moment you recognize that your unconscious is re-running a negative loop. It's sneaky and will stay in habitual patterns, like worry, unless you retrain it. *Easy?* No, but practice will garner results. The first step is to recognize when it's happening. Then ask yourself, What do I really want to feel now? And move toward that feeling. Practice, practice, *practice*.

You need to keep your eyes on where you want to be and keep steering toward it. You have the power to change you and the way you respond to the world around you. That's perhaps what's really meant by the Jane Roberts quote, "You create your own reality."

Take a leap—right now—right past what seems like your "reality"—right past your inner critic, biases from culture or family, your habits, opinions, ideals, dislikes, shadow, and light and just stop the internal noise for a time and Be genuinely and absolutely happy. Bring that sensation out of your own imagination or out of the moth balls of a past experience. Give this gift to yourself several times a day. Anything that you're going through will be a thousand times improved.

Our camouflage, our masks, become so convenient and so completely habitual that sometimes we believe them ourselves. We literally forget who we are. Driven by the quest to just keep ahead of our debts and our debtors, our trespasses and our trespassers, it becomes a challenge to genuinely answer the question "What do you want?" Please explore for yourself the value difference in living a successful life and living a significant life. It's your life—now what do you want in this life?

What gets you fired up? What will your legacy be? What does your life stand for? Dr. Peter Marshall, a U.S. Senate Chaplain said, "...unless we stand for something, we shall fall for anything."[2] We leave ourselves vulnerable to all manner of potential negative influences when we lose track of our selves. These questions may sound huge, but they are fundamental to your life and are underlying sources of stress every bit as pervasive as family, work, and financial pressures. You can't answer these questions if your mind is racing with a hundred thoughts. You need to Be clear.

You now have shiny new tools which you can put between yourself and the madness. Use the Stop Technique several times throughout your day. Use deep breathing or meditation morning and evening to balance your day. Stretch your body to relieve some tension every day. Write out your frustrations, let loose an Inner Scream. Exercise at least three times weekly. Eat some amazing, flavorful, nutritious food, and get some sleep!

Sometimes, the sole action that you can take is to heal your attitude toward self and life. Embrace the philosophy that "this is the only body that I have and I want to treat it in a loving and respectful way." Then, if you can really feel and believe this, you will just naturally begin to eat better, exercise more, learn to handle your stresses, and have a new and different approach to your life.

You're here—why not make some better choices? Find ways to make positive changes in your environment beyond air, food, and water. Try new friendships, lifestyles, communities, work, and cultural conditions. All are essential. Your reaction to your environment is the key to your health.

When you heal your wounds, you really do assist in the healing of others; you transform the consciousness in your family and in the world—maybe in small ways—maybe in large ways. Consider the butterfly effect attributed to Edward Norton Lorenz, mathematician and meteorologist, wherein the flapping of a butterfly's wings in South America could affect the weather in Texas; meaning that the tiniest influence on one part of a system can have a huge effect on another part.[3] The dramatic transformation of the butterfly is Divine proof that we can have a second life. You are that butterfly.

Breathe, slowly and deeply, smile and remember who you are...and get started.

Appendix

SUPPLEMENT	NOTES
Vitamin C (crystalline powder)	Important in helping to reduce and balance blood sugar, as well as immune support, cell function, and restoration. Food sources include green peppers, grapefruit, and oranges.
Vitamin K2	Synthesized in the intestines, increases menaquinone intake and may reduce the development of insulin resistance and thereby offer protection against Type-2 diabetes. Beneficial for bone health. Mainly found in fermented foods such as organic kefir, ripe cheese, yogurt, and a fermented soy food known as natto.
Vitamin D3 (cholecalciferol)	Necessary for overall health—immune system support, reducing inflammation, and boosting mood. Not obtaining enough of this important nutrient can leave you open to developing a number of health conditions. Have your levels checked. *See additional info on pages 163 and 164.*
Vitamin E (mixed tocopherols)	Potent antioxidant, and also important in assisting with reduction and balancing blood sugar. Food sources include leafy green vegetables, nuts, and seeds.
Coenzyme Q10 as ubiquinol	Another essential antioxidant that also increases cellular energy production, and free radical elimination.

Alpha-lipoic Acid	Powerful antioxidant proven to reduce blood sugar significantly. It also can be effective for diabetic nerve damage.
Calcium and Magnesium	Help with glucose metabolism and healthy bone formation. Play an essential role in blood clotting, muscle contraction, and nerve impulse transmission. Studies show that they help with relaxation. Food sources include collard greens, broccoli, and spinach.
B-complex Vitamins	As the name implies, this blend of vitamins works together to support brain and body systems that cope with stressors: B1 (thiamine) breaks down sugars in the diet and is in charge of immune and adrenal gland function and the manufacture of neurotransmitters; B2 (riboflavin) and B3 (niacin) promotes vibrant energy production; B5 (pantothenic acid) is required for adrenal stress hormone production, as well as appropriate energy and immune function.
Chromium	Benefits in utilization and control of carbohydrates and protein in the body. Very important for proper sugar metabolism. Also increases healthy muscle and tissue growth.
Omega-3 Fish Oil	Reduces inflammation, improves insulin sensitivity, and lowers cholesterol.
N-Acetyl Cysteine	An amino acid and effective antioxidant and cell detoxifier, it plays an important role in the manufacture of glutathione, and is crucial to neutralize free radicals and to cleanse.

L-Arginine	An amino acid that assists in cardiovascular function. Shown to relax blood vessels for smoother and faster transport of blood to and from the heart. Supports both healthy blood pressure and bodily processes.
L-Carnitine	Another amino acid that permits the body to burn more fat, save more glycogen, and boosts stamina.

Vitamin D3

Because your body only makes vitamin D3 when your skin is exposed to sunlight, you may be at risk of deficiency. If you live in a northern hemisphere, this location prevents you from getting enough sun (and therefore vitamin D3) to begin with, especially during winter. *And* you're probably not eating enough of the few natural dietary sources of vitamin D3—fatty, wild, cold-water fish like mackerel, halibut, herring, sardines, and cod liver oil. Plus, as we age, our skin naturally produces less vitamin D3. The fact is that the average 70-year-old person creates only 25 percent of the vitamin D3 that a 20 year-old does. Also, people with darker skin complexions naturally produce less vitamin D3.

Vitamin D3's anti–inflammatory effects cross a wide variety of health conditions including diabetes, hypertension, and psoriasis. Vitamin D3 also helps regulate your immune system activity, which when working properly, will prevent any excessive or prolonged inflammatory response.

Immune cells, specifically your active T-cells, have built-in receptors for vitamin D3. This is a critical factor because they respond to auto-immune diseases, which includes diabetes, rheumatoid arthritis, multiple sclerosis, irritable bowel diseases (Crohn's and ulcerative colitis all have a T-cell component of inflammation). Vitamin D3 deficiency has even been linked to breast, colon, prostate, and ovarian cancer.

Obesity and surplus weight-gain is a vitamin D3 matter too. Researchers from Kaiser Permanete Center for Health Research in Portland, Oregon, did a five-year study involving more than 4,600 women (age 65 and above). The study revealed that those with insufficient amounts of vitamin D3 in their blood gained two pounds more than those with sufficient levels. "Nearly 80 percent of women in our study had insufficient levels of vitamin D3," concluded study author Erin LeBlanc, MD.[1]

But before you run out to buy some oral vitamin D3, it would be very prudent to monitor your vitamin D3 blood levels regularly through blood testing with your doctor.

Chlorella

Chlorella is considered a whole food, one that is a complete protein. Amazingly, it contains all of the essential B vitamins, as well as vitamins E and C. In addition, chlorella contains all of the major minerals including zinc and iron. *Impressive?* It reportedly balances the pH levels in your body. Another of the chlorella benefits is that it helps the body to break down metallic toxins. These toxins include mercury, cadmium, and lead among others. Not only does this amazing food boost your immune system, it also:

» Accelerates healing and protects against radiation.
» Aids you in promoting optimal blood pressure.
» Cleanses key elimination systems like your bowel, liver, and blood.
» Promotes growth and repair of your tissues.
» Aids your body in processing more oxygen.
» Supports elimination of molds in your body.
» Helps purify your blood and clean away toxins.

With all of that, chlorella benefits include major assistance in the prevention of degenerative diseases, relief from arthritis pain, and has been reported to help in losing weight and aid in Candida albicans treatment.

Notes

Chapter 1: What Makes Us Sick?

1. Bruce Lipton, *The Biology of Belief* (California: Hay House, 2007), 148.

2. John Cairns, J. Overbaugh, and S. Miller, "The Origin of Mutants." *Nature* 335 (1988): 142–145. (This was first major paper on "adaptive" mutations, that is, mutations that are not random.)

3. F. Marotta, Y. Naito, F. Padrini, X. Xuewei, S. Jain, V. Soresi, L. Zhou, R. Catanzaro, K. Zhong, A. Polimeni, D.H. Chui., "Redox Balance Signaling in Occupational Stress: Modification by Nutraceutical Intervention." *Journal of Biological Regulators and Homeostatic Agents* 25(2) (April–June 2011): 221–9.

4. Kathleen Fackelmann, "Stress Can Ravage the Body, Unless the Mind Says No," *USA Today* March 21, 2005.

Chapter 2: Stress: The Equal Opportunity Assassin

1. Department of Health and Human Services, Federal Occupational Health annual Stress Awareness Month, *www.foh.hhs.gov/dbdmarketing/nsam.html*.

2. Center for Disease Prevention, National Center for Health Statistics, *www.cdc.gov/nchs/fastats/diabetes.htm*

3. E. Carlsson, A. Frostell, J. Ludvigsson, M. Faresjo, "Psychological Stress in Children May Alter the Immune Response." *The*

Journal of Immunology 192(5) (2014): 2071, doi: 10.4049/jimmunol.1301713.

4.   Florent Elefteriou, J. Preston, et al., "Stimulation of Host Bone Marrow Stromal Cells by Sympathetic Nerves Promotes Breast Cancer Bone Metastasis in Mice." *PLOS Biology*, 17 (2012): doi: 10.1371/journal.pbio.1001363

5.   Lauri Nummenmaa, Enrico Glerean, et al., "Bodily maps of emotions." *Proceedings of the National Academy of Sciences* 111(2) (2014): 646–651, doi:10.1073/pnas.1321664111; cf "How emotions are mapped in the body." *ScienceDaily* 31 (2013).

6.   Harold E. Sconiers, "Health Benefits From Smiling." LiveStrong Website blog, 24 October 2013.

7.   Marc G. Berman, John Jonides, and Stephen Kaplan, "The Cognitive Benefits of Interacting with Nature," University of Michigan, *www.umich.edu/~jlabpsyc/pdf/2008_2.pdf*

8.   Amy Gallo, "Turning Stress into an Asset." *Harvard Business Review* 28 (June 2011).

9.   Shawn Achor, *The Happiness Advantage*. Random House (2010).

Chapter 3: Breathe Your Way to Better Mental and Physical Health

1.   Debra A. Werntz, R.G. Bickford, and D. Shannahoff-Khalsa, "Selective hemispheric stimulation by unilateral forced nostril breathing." *Human Neurobiology* (1987).

2.   Meesha Joshi, Shirley Telles, "Immediate effects of right and left nostril breathing on verbal and spatial scores," *Indian Journal of Physiology and Pharmacology* 52 (April–June 2008): 197–200.

3.   Dr. Candace Pert, *Molecules of Emotion: The Science Behind Mind-Body Medicine*. (New York: Simon & Schuster, 1999).

4. A. Stancak, Jr. and M. Kuna, "EEG Changes During Forced Alternate Nostril Breathing" International Journal of Psychophysiology 1 (1994): 75–9

5. Ibid.

Chapter 4: Eat, Drink and Be Healthy (Food as Information)

1. Annika Rosengren, et al. "Stressful life events, social support, and mortality in men born in 1933." *British Medical Journal* (1993): 1102–1105.

2. Maarit Korkeila, et al. "Predictors of major weight gain in adult Finns: stress, life satisfaction and personality traits." *International Journal of Obesity & Related Metabolic Disorders* 22.10 (1998).

3. Jeremy D. Akers, Rachel A. Cornett, Jyoti S. Savla, Kevin P. Davy, et al., "Daily Self-Monitoring of Body Weight, Step Count, Fruit/Vegetable Intake, and Water Consumption: A Feasible and Effective Long-Term Weight Loss Maintenance Approach." *Journal of the Academy of Nutrition and Dietetics* 112(5): 685–692.

4. Edward Howell, *Enzyme Nutrition: The Food Enzyme Concept.* (New York: Penguin, 1985).

5. Robert G. Maunder, "Evidence that stress contributes to inflammatory bowel disease: evaluation, synthesis, and future directions." *Inflammatory bowel diseases* 11.6 (2005): 600–608.

6. Candace B. Pert, *Molecules of Emotion: Why You Feel the Way You Feel.* (New York: Simon and Schuster, 1997).

7. National Cancer Institute, Surveillance, Epidemiology and End Results Program, Fact Sheet Pancreas; cf GI Health Website *www.gihealth.com/html/education/pancreaticCancer.html*

8. Sarah Wild, et al. "Global prevalence of diabetes estimates for the year 2000 and projections for 2030." *Diabetes Care* 27.5 (2004): 1047–1053.

9. Robert M. Russell, MD, "Gastric Hypochlorhydria and Achlorhydria in Older Adults" *Journal of the American Medical Association* 278 (1997): 1659, doi:10.1001/jama.1997.

10. Mitchel H. Katz, MD, "Failing the Acid Test." *Archives of Internal Medicine* 170(9) (2010); cf *www.archinternmed.com*.

11. Harold McGee. *On Food and Cooking: The Science and Lore of the Kitchen.* (New York: Simon and Schuster, 2007).

12. Dr. Joseph Mercola, "How to Starve Cancer Out of Your Body —Avoid These Top 4 Cancer-Feeding Foods" transcript of video: Dr. Joseph Mercola Interviews Dr. Christine Horner, YouTube.

13. "Harvard Nurses' Health Study" *www.channing.harvard.edu/nhs*.

14. Mary Enig and Sally Fallon, *Nourishing Traditions*, (Lanham, Ma.: New Trends Publishing, Inc., 2001).

15. C. Danielson, J.L. Lyon, M Egger, G.K. Goodenough, "Hip Fractures and Fluoridation in Utah's Elderly Population." *Journal of the American Medical Association* 268(6) (1992): 746–748, doi:10.1001/jama.1992.03490060078027.

16. B. Lawrence Riggs, MD, Stephen F. Hodgson, MD, et al., "Effect of Fluoride Treatment on the Fracture Rate in Postmenopausal Women with Osteoporosis." New England Journal of Medicine 322 (1990): 802–809, doi: 10.1056/NEJM199003223221203.

17. Malcolm W. Browne, "Rat Study Reignites Dispute On Fluoride." *New York Times*, 13 March 1990.

18. John Yiamouyiannis, et al., "Cancer mortality and fluoridation." *The Lancet* 311.8056 (1978): 150–151.

19. John Yiamouyiannis, "Fluoride the Aging Factor: How to Recognize and Avoid the Devastating Effects of Fluoride," *Health Action Periodical* 3 (1993).

Chapter 5: Stretching

1. Cedric X. Bryant, PhD, "When is the best time to stretch?" *Fellow American College of Sports Medicine* 5 January 2010.

2. Edmund Jacobson, "Progressive relaxation." (1938).

Chapter 6: Movement

1. Transcript of a Special Interview with Phil Campbell by Dr. Joseph Mercola *http://mercola.fileburst.com/PDF/ExpertInterviewTranscripts/InterviewPhilCampbell.pdf*

2. University of Copenhagen, "30 minutes of daily exercise does the trick: Same effect in half the time." *ScienceDaily*, 22 (2012).

3. Mark Peterson, PhD and Paul M. Gordon, PhD, MPH, "Resistance Exercise for the Aging Adult: Clinical Implications and Prescription Guidelines." *The American Journal of Medicine* 124 (2011): 194–198.

4. Katherine Hobson, "How to Avoid Losing Muscle as You Age," *U.S. News and World Report*, 4 September 2008.

5. D. Paddon-Jones, T. Brock Symons, et al., "A moderate serving of high-quality protein maximally stimulates skeletal muscle protein synthesis in young and elderly subjects." *Journal of the American Dietetic Association* 109.9 (2009): 1582–1586.

6. Centers for Disease Control—The National Health and Nutrition Examination Survey (NHANES) Archive *www.cdc.gov/nchs/nhanes.htm*

7. P.T. Katzmarzyk, "Sedentary behaviour and life expectancy in the USA: a cause-deleted life table analysis." *British Medical Journal* 2 (2012), doi: e000828. doi:10.1136/bmjopen-2012-000828

8. Chad Kerksick and Darryn Willoughby, "The antioxidant role of glutathione and N–acetyl–cysteine supplements and exercise-induced oxidative stress." *Journal of International Society and Sports Nutrition* 2.2 (2005): 38–44.

9. American Physiological Society (APS). "Exercise could fortify immune system against future cancers." *ScienceDaily*. 10 October 2012.

10. Ibid.

Chapter 7: Anxiety (or Dance With the Elephants)

1. J.A. Bargh, M. Chen, and L. Burrows, "Automaticity of Social Behavior: Direct Effects of Trait Construct and Stereotype-Activation on Action." *Journal of Personality and Social Psychology* 71 (1996): 230–244.

2. *www.goodreads.com/author/quotes/3503.Maya_Angelou*

3. Octavia E. Butler, *Parable of the Sower*. (New York: Grand Central Publishing, 2000).

4. James W. Pennebaker, *Writing to Heal: A Guided Journal for Recovering from Trauma & Emotional Upheaval*. (New York: New Harbinger Publications, Inc, 2004.)

Chapter 9: Brainwave Entrainment

1. Herber Benson, "The Relaxation Response" (New York: William Paperbacks, 2000).

Noam Sobel, et al., "Humans Can Learn New Infor- ng Sleep." *Nature Neuroscience* (2012), doi: 10.1038/

Chapter 10: Sleep (Get More!)

1. R.E. Roberts and H.T. Duong. "The prospective association between sleep deprivation and depression among adolescents." *Sleep* 37 (2014): 239–244.

2. Dorothy Foltz-Gray, "7 Surprising Health Benefits of Sleep." *Lifescript* (2013).

3. Ibid.

4. Christian Benedict, et al., "Acute sleep deprivation increases serum levels of neuron-specific enolase (NSE) and S100 calcium binding protein B (S-100B) in healthy young men." *Sleep* 37.1 (2013): 195–198.

5. Francesco Cappuccio, et al., "Gender-specific associations of short sleep duration with prevalent and incident hypertension the Whitehall II study." *Hypertension* 50.4 (2007): 693–700.

6. Dorothy Foltz-Gray, "7 Surprising Health Benefits of Sleep." *Lifescript* (2013).

7. Ibid.

8. Josée Savard, et al., "Randomized study on the efficacy of cognitive-behavioral therapy for insomnia secondary to breast cancer, part II: Immunologic effects." *Journal of Clinical Oncology* 23.25 (2005): 6097–6106.

9. University of Helsinki. "New links between sleep deprivation, immune system discovered." *ScienceDaily*. 23 October 2013.

10. Vilma Aho, et al., "Partial Sleep Restriction Activates Immune Response-Related Gene Expression Pathways: Experimental and Epidemiological Studies in Humans." *Public Library of Science* 8.10 (2013).

11. Ibid.

12. Ibid.

13. Ibid.

14. Ibid.

15. Mauro Marcel Mattos, "Machine Biological Clock: Exploring the Time Dimension in an Organic-Based Operating System."

16. Ines Wilhelm, Jan Born, et al., "Is the cortisol awakening rise a response to awakening?" *Psychoneuroendocrinology* 32, no. 4 (2007): 358–366.

17. Baylor College of Medicine. "Heart beats to the rhythm of a circadian clock." *ScienceDaily*. 22 February 2012.

18. Mary A. Carskadon and William C. Dement. "Cumulative effects of sleep restriction on daytime sleepiness." *Psychophysiology* 18.2 (1981): 107–113.

19. Kim Youngsoo, Fred Turek, Aaron D. Laposky, et al., "Repeated sleep restriction in rats leads to homeostatic and allostatic responses during recovery sleep." *Proceedings of the National Academy of Sciences* 104.25 (2007): 10697–10702.

20. Ibid.

21. Ibid.

22. Daniel Cohen, et al., "Uncovering Residual Effects of Chronic Sleep Loss on Human Performance." *Science Translational Medicine* 2 (2010), doi: 10.1126/scitranslmed.3000458: PMCID: PMC2892834

23. Lawrence Epstein and Steve Mardon, "The Harvard Medical School Guide to a Good Night's Sleep." *Harvard Medical School Guides* (2006)

24. Robert Meadows, "The 'negotiated night': an embodied conceptual framework for the sociological study of sleep." *The Sociological Review* 53.2 (2005): 240–254.

25. U.S. National Sleep Foundation.

26. National Association of Home Builders.

27. University of Chicago Medical Center. "Even your fat cells need sleep, according to new research." *ScienceDaily* 15 October 2012.

28. Ibid.

29. Ibid.

30. Ibid.

31. Ibid.

32. Ibid.

33. Johanni Hansen, "Working Nights Associated With Increased Risk of Breast Cancer" *Journal of the National Cancer Institute* 93 (2001): 1511 doi:10.1093/jnci/93.20.1511-b.

34. Mary Bellis, "Humphry Davy an English chemist invented the first electric light." *About.com/Inventors*.

35. Hattar, Samer. et al. "Aberrant light directly impairs mood and learning through melanopsin-expressing neurons." Nature. 2012 Nov 22;491(7425):594-8. doi: 10.1038/nature11673. Epub 2012 Nov 14.

36. Ibid.

Conclusion

1. "A Poet's Advice to Students" in *E. E. Cummings, A Miscellany*, edited by George James Firmage (1958): 13.

2. P. Marshall P., "Senate chaplain, prayer offered at the opening of the session." Senate Document 20 (1949).

3. T.N. Palmer, "Edward Norton Lorenz 23 May 1917–16 April 2008." *Biographical Memoirs of Fellows of the Royal Society* (2009).

Appendix

1. Erin S. LeBlanc, MD, MPH, Joanne H. Rizzo, MPA, Kathryn L. Pedula, MS, et al., "The Endocrine Society's Clinical Guidelines for the Evaluation, Treatment and Prevention of Vitamin D Deficiency." *Journal of Clinical Endocrinology & Metabolism* 96 (2011): 1911–1930.

Bibliography

Chapter 1: What Makes Us Sick?

Cairns, John, J. Overbaugh, and S. Miller. "The Origin of Mutants" *Nature* 335 (1988): 142–145.

Crabbe, J.C. and T.J. Phillips. "Mother Nature Meets Mother Nurture." *Nature Neuroscience* 6 (2003): 440–442.

Crum A.J., P. Salovey, and S. Achor. "Rethinking stress: the role of mindsets in determining the stress response." *Journal of Personality and Social Psychology.* 104 vol. 4 (2013):716–33.

Dhabhar F.S., W.B. Malarkey, E. Neri E, and B.S. McEwen. "Stress-induced redistribution of immune cells—from barracks to boulevards to battlefields: a tale of three hormones." *Psychoneuroendocrinology* 37: (2012) 1345–68.

Fraga, M.F., et al. "Epigenetic differences arise during the lifetime of monozygotic twins." *Proceedings of the National Academy of Sciences* 102 (2005):10604-10609.

Gershon, Michael D., MD. *The Second Brain—The Scientific Bases of Gut Instinct.* New York: Harper Collins, 1998.

Jablonka, E. and M. J. Lamb. *Evolution in Four Dimensions: Genetic, Epigenetic, Behavioral, and Symbolic Variation in the History of Life.* UK: Bradford Books, 2005.

Marotta, F., Y. Naito, F. Padrini, X. Xuewei, S. Jain, V. Soresi, L. Zhou, R. Catanzaro, K. Zhong, A. Polimeni, D.H. Chui. "Redox Balance Signaling in Occupational Stress: Modification by Nutraceutical Intervention." *Journal of Biological Regulators and Homeostatic Agents* 25 (2011): 221–9.

Pauling, Linus, Phd. *How to Live Longer and Feel Better.* Portland: Oregon State University Press, 2006.

Pert, Candace, Dr. *Molecules of Emotion: The Science Behind Mind-Body Medicine.* New York: Simon & Schuster, 1999.

Powell, K. "It's the Ecology, Stupid!" *Nature* 435 (2005): 268–271.

Pray, Leslie. "Epigenetics: Genome, Meet Your Environment." *The Scientist* 18 (2004): 14.

Chapter 2: Stress: The Equal Opportunity Assassin

Achor, Shawn. *The Happiness Advantage.* New York: Random House, 2010.

Berman, Marc G., John Jonides, and Stephen Kaplan. "The Cognitive Benefits of Interacting with Nature." University of Michigan, *www.umich. edu/~jlabpsyc/pdf/2008_2.pdf*

Calvo, Manuel G., L. Nummenmaa, and Pedro Avero. "Recognition advantage of happy faces in extrafoveal vision: Featural and affective processing." *Visual Cognition* 18.9 (2010): 1274–1297.

Campbell, J. Preston, Matthew R. Karolak, Yun Ma, Daniel S. Perrien, S. Kathryn Masood-Campbell, Niki L. Penner, Steve A. Munoz, Andries Zijlstra, Xiangli Yang, Julie A. Sterling, and Florent Elefteriou. "Stimulation of Host Bone Marrow Stromal Cells by Sympathetic Nerves Promotes Breast Cancer Bone Metastasis in Mice." *Public Library of Science*, July 17, 2012, doi: 10.1371/journal.pbio.1001363.

Disease & Emotion Relationship *www.cdc.gov/ncipc/pub-res/pdf/childhood_stress.pdf*

Epel, E.S., B. McEwen, T. Seeman, et al. "Stress and Body Shape: Stress-Induced Cortisol Secretion is Consistently Greater among Women with Central Fat." *Psychosomatic Medicine* 62 (2000):623–632.

Finkel, T. "Oxidants, Oxidative Stress and the Biology of Ageing." *Nature* 408 (2000): 239–47.

Heart Attack Statistics. New England Journal of Medicine, July, 22 1999.

Holmes, T.H. and R.H. Rahe. "The Social Readjustment Rating Scale" *J. Psychosom. Res.* 11 vol. 2 (1967): 213–8.

Kahn, P.H., Jr. *The Human Relationship With Nature: Development and Culture.* Cambridge, Mass.: MIT Press, 1999.

Kahn, Jr., P.H., Rachel L. Severson, and Jolina H. Ruckert. "The Human Relation With Nature and Technological Nature." University of Washington, *http:// depts.washington.edu/hints/publications/Human_Relation_Technological_Nature.pdf.*

Kirby E.D., S.E. Muroy, W.G. Sun, D. Covarrubia, M.J. Leong, L.A. Barchas, and D. Kaufer. "Acute stress enhances adult rat hippocampal neurogenesis and activation of newborn neurons via secreted astrocytic FGF2." *Elife.* (2013), doi: 10.7554/eLife.00362. Print 2013.

Morrow, J.D. "Quantification of Isoprostanes as Indices of Oxidant Stress and the Risk of Atherosclerosis in Humans." *Arteriosclerosis, Thrombosis, and Vascular Biology* 25 vol. 2 (2005): 279–86.

Nummenmaa, L. E. Glerean, R. Hari, J. K. Hietanen. "Bodily Maps of Emotions." *Proceedings of the National Academy of Sciences* (2013), doi, *http://dx.doi. org/10.1073/pnas.1321664111*

Chapter 3: Breathe Your Way to Better Mental & Physical Health

Amen, Daniel G.and Lisa C. Routh. *Healing Anxiety and Depression.* New York: Berkley Trade, 2004.

Jerath, R., J.W. Edry, V.A. Barnes, and V. Jerath. "Physiology of long pranayamic breathing: Neural respiratory elements may provide a mechanism that explains how slow deep breathing shifts the autonomic nervous system." *Medical Hypothesis* 67 (2006): 566–571. Ritz, T. and W.T.

Pal, G.K., S. Velkumary, and Madanmohan. "Effect of Short-term Practice of Breathing Exercises on Autonomic Functions in Normal Human Volunteers." *Indian Journal of Medical Research*, 120 (2004): 115–121. Roth. "Behavioral Intervention in Asthma." *Behavior Modification* 27 (2003): 710–73.

Sovik, R. "The Science of Breathing—The Yogic View." *Progress in Brain Research.* 122 (2000): 491–505.

Stancák Jr., A. and M. Kuna. "Changes During Forced Alternate Nostril Breathing." International Journal of Psychophysiology. 18 vol. 1 (1994): 75–9.

Werntz, D.A., R.G. Bickford, and D. Shannahoff-Khalsa. "Selective hemispheric stimulation by unilateral forced nostril breathing." *Human Neurobiology* 6 (1987): 165–71.

Chapter 4: Eat, Drink, and Be Healthy (Food as Information)

Ambrosone, C.B. and L. Tang. "Cruciferous Vegetable Intake and Cancer Prevention: Role of Nutrigenetics." *Cancer Prevention* 2 (2009): 298–300.

Angeloni, C., E. Leoncini, M. Malaguti, et al. "Modulation Of Phase II Enzymes by Sulforaphane: Implications for its Cardio-protective Potential." Journal of Agricultural Food Chemistry. 24 (2009): 5615–22.

Bourre, J.M. "Dietary Omega-3 Fatty Acids and Psychiatry: Mood, Behaviour, Stress, Depression, Dementia and Aging." Journal of Nutrition, Health, and Aging. 9 (2005): 31–8.

Harvard Nurses' Health Study *www.channing.harvard.edu/nhs/*.

Howell, Edward. *Enzyme Nutrition: The Food Enzyme Concept.* New York: Penguin, 1985.

Higdon, J.V., B. Delage, D.E. Williams, et al. "Cruciferous Vegetables and Human Cancer Risk: Epidemiologic Evidence and Mechanistic Basis." Pharmacological Research 55 (2007): 224–236.

Hyman, Dr. Mark. *The Blood Sugar Solution.* New York: Little, Brown and Company, 2012.

Konturek, P.C., T. Brzozowski, and S.J. Konturek. "Stress and the Gut: Pathophysiology, Clinical Consequences, Diagnostic Approach and Treatment Options." *Journal of Physiology and Pharmacology* 62 (2011): 591–599.

Lyte, M., L. Vulchanova, D.R. Brown. "Stress at the intestinal surface: catecholamines and mucosa-bacteria interactions." *Cell and Tissue Research* 343 (2011): 23–32.

Bibliography

Marotta, F., G.S. Mao, T. Liu, D.H. Chui, A. Lorenzetti, Y. Xiao, P. Marandola. "Anti-inflammatory and Neuroprotective Effect of a Phytoestrogen Compound on Rat Microglia." *Annals of the New York Academy of Sciences* 1089 (2006): 276–281.

Medina, M.A. "Glutamine and Cancer." *Journal of Nutrition* 131 (2001): 2539S-42S.

Mercola, Joseph and Kendra Pearsall. "Take Control of Your Health." *www.prod ucts.mercola.com/take-control*

Mullenix, Phyllis, et al. "Neurotoxicity of Sodium Fluoride in Rats." *Neurotoxicology and Teratology* 17 (1995): 169–177.

Novak, N., L. Björck, K.W., C. Giang, L. Heden-Ståhl, and A. Wilhelmsen. "Perceived stress and incidence of Type 2 diabetes: a 35-year follow-up study of middle-aged Swedish men." *Diabetic Medicine* 30 (2013): e8.

Paddon-Jones, D., E. Westman, R. Mattes, et al. "Protein, Weight Management, and Satiety." *American Journal of Clinical Nutrition* 87 (2008): 1558S–1561S.

Perica, M.M. and I. Delas. "Essential Fatty Acids and Psychiatric Disorders." *Nutrition in Clinical Practice* 26 (2011): 409–25.

Pert, Candace B. *Molecules of Emotion: Why You Feel the Way You Feel.* New York: Simon and Schuster, 1997.

Proton-Pump Inhibitors *www.ncbi.nlm.nih.gov/pubmed/20458079*

Rios, A., N. Delgado-Casado, C. Cruz-Teno, E.M. Yubero-Serrano, F. Tinahones, M.D. Malagon, F. Perez-Jimenez, J. Lopez-Miranda. "Mediterranean Diet Reduces Senescence-Associated Stress in Endothelial Cells" (2011).

Stecher, P., et al. *The Merck Index of Chemicals and Drugs.* Rahway, N.J.: Merck & Company, 1960.

Stough, C., A. Scholey, J. Lloyd, J. Spong, S. Myers, and L.A. Downey. "The Effect of 90 day Administration of a High Dose Vitamin B-Complex on Work Stress." Human Psychopharmacology 8 (2011).

Talha, Jawaid, Deepa Shukla, and Jaiendra Verma. "Anti-Inflammatory Activity of The Plants Used in Traditional Medicines." *International Journal of Biomedical Research,* doi: 10.7439/ijbr.v2i4.102.

Tang, L., G.R. Zirpoli, K. Guru, et al. "Consumption of Raw Cruciferous Vegetables is Inversely Associated with Bladder Cancer Risk." *Cancer Research* 67 (2007): 3569–73.

Tarozzi, A., F. Morroni, A. Merlicco, et al. "Sulforaphane as an Inducer of Glutathione Prevents Oxidative Stress-Induced Cell Death in a Dopaminergic-Like Neuroblastoma Cell Line." Journal of Neurochemistry. 111(2009): 1161–71.

Wang, G, et al. "Research on Intelligence Quotient of 4-7 year-old Children in a District with a High Level of Fluoride." *Endemic Diseases Bulletin* 11 (1996): 60-62.

Yehuda, S., S. Rabinovitz, D.I. Mostofsky. "Mixture of Essential Fatty Acids Lowers Test Anxiety." *Nutrition and Neuroscience* 8 (2005): 265–7.

Zhao, L.B., et al. "Effect of High Fluoride Water Supply on Children's Intelligence." *Fluoride*, 29 (1996): 190–192.

Chapter 5: Stretching

Jacobson, Edmund. *Progressive Relaxation: A Physiological & Clinical Investigation of Muscular States & Their Significance in Psychology & Medical Practice.* Chicago: University of Chicago, 1974.

Luthe, W. and J.H. Schultz. *Autogenic Therapy.* London: The British Autogenic Society, 2001.

Chapter 6: Movement

Campbell, Phil. *Ready, Set, Go!* New York: Pristine Publishers, Inc., 2007.

Epel, E.S., Blackburn, E.H., J. Lin, F.S. Dhabhar, N.E. Adler, J.D. Morrow, R.M. Cawthon. "Accelerated Telomere Shortening in Response to Life Stress." *Proceedings of the National Academy of Sciences.* 101 (2004): 17312–5.

Lin, J., E. Epel, E. Blackburn. "Telomeres and Lifestyle Factors: Roles in Cellular Aging." *Mutation Research.* (2011).

Nelson, Miriam E. and Sarah Wernick, PhD. *Strong Women Stay Young.* New York: Bantam Books, 2005.

Nuttall, S., U. Martin, A. Sinclair, M. Kendall. "Glutathione: in Sickness and in Health." *The Lancet* 351(1998): 645–646.

Paddon-Jones, D. and B. Rasmussen. "Dietary Protein Recommendations and the Prevention of Sarcopenia: Protein, Amino Acid Metabolism and Therapy." *Current Opinion in Clinical Nutrition and Metabolic Care* 12 (2009): 86–90.

Peterson, Mark D. and Paul M. Gordon. "Resistance Exercise for the Aging Adult: Clinical Implications and Prescription Guidelines." *The American Journal of Medicine* 124 (2011): 194.

Rosenkilde, M., P. L. Auerbach, M.H. Reichkendler, T. Ploug, B.M. Stallknecht, and A. Sjodin. "Body fat loss and compensatory mechanisms in response to different doses of aerobic exercise—a randomized controlled trial in over weight sedentary males." *AJP: Regulatory, Integrative and Comparative Physiology.* (2012).

Chapter 7: Anxiety (or Dance with the Elephants)

Bargh, J.A., M. Chen, L. Burrows. "Automaticity of Social Behavior: Direct Effects of Trait Construct and Stereotype-Activation on Action." *Journal of Personality and Social Psychology* 71 (1996): 230–244.

Cyphert, Dale. "Managing Stage Fright." *www.cba.uni.edu/buscomm/Presentations/stagefright.html*

Pennebaker, James W. *Writing to Heal: A Guided Journal for Recovering from Trauma & Emotional Upheaval.* Oakland, Calif.: New Harbinger Publications, 2004.

Rudd, Melanie, Jennifer Aaker, and Kathleen Vohs. "Awe Expands People's Perception of Time, Alters Decision Making, and Enhances Well-Being." *Psychological Science* (2012).

Chapter 8: Meditation

Delmonte, M.M. "Electro-cortical Activity and Related Phenomena Associated with Meditation Practice." *International Journal of Neuroscience* 24 (1984): 217–231.

Jevning, R., R.K. Wallace, and M. Beidenbach. "The Physiology of Meditation: A review. A Wakeful Hypnometabolic Integrated Response." *Neuroscience and Behavioral Reviews* 16 (1992): 415–424.

Sabourin, M.E., S.E. Cutcomb, H.J. Crawford, and K. Pribram. "EEG Correlates of Hypnotic Susceptibility and Hypnotic Trance: Spectral Analysis and Coherence." *International Journal of Psychophysiology* 10 (1990): 125-142.

Chapter 9: Brainwave Entrainment

Anat Arzi, Limor Shedlesky, Mor Ben-Shaul, Khitam Nasser, Arie Oksenberg, Ilana S. Hairston, and Noam Sobel. "Humans Can Learn New Information During Sleep." *Nature Neuroscience* (2012).

Antony, James W., Eric W. Gobel, Justin K. O'Hare, Paul J. Reber, and Ken A. Paller. "Cued Memory Reactivation During Sleep Influences Skill Learning." *Nature Neuroscience* (2012).

Cai, D.J.; S.A. Mednick, E.M. Harrison, J.C. Kanady, and S.C. Mednick. "REM, not Incubation, Improves Creativity by Priming Associative Networks." *Proceedings of the National Academy of Sciences* 106 (2009): 10130–10134.

Guilfoyle, G. and D. Carbone. "The Facilitation of Attention Utilizing Therapeutic Sounds." Presented at the New York State Association of Day Service Providers Symposium, October 18, 1996, Albany, New York.

Kaufman, Marc. "Meditation Gives Brain a Charge, Study Finds." *The Washington Post.* January 3, 2005. Retrieved May 3, 2010.

Lutz A., L.L. Greischar, N.B. Rawlings, M. Ricard, R.J. Davidson. "Long-term Meditators Self-Induce High Amplitude Gamma Synchrony During Mental Practice." *Proceedings of the National Academy of Sciences* 101: (2005): 16369–16373.

Bibliography

Melloni, L., C. Molina, M. Pena, D. Torres, W. Singer, E. Rodriguez. "Synchronization of Neural Activity Across Cortical Areas Correlates with Conscious Perception." *Journal of Neuroscience* 27 (2007): 2858–65.

O'Nuallain, Sean. "Zero Power and Selflessness: What Meditation and Conscious Perception Have in Common." *Journal: Cognitive Sciences* 4 (2009).

Singer, W. and C.M. Gray. "Visual feature Integration and the Temporal Correlation Hypothesis." *Annual Review of Neuroscience* 18 (1995): 555–586.

Smith, J.C., J.T. Marsh, and W.S. Brown. "Far-field Recorded Frequency-following Responses: Evidence for the Locus of Brainstem Sources." *Electroencephalography and Clinical Neurophysiology* 39 (1975): 465–472.

Smith, J.C., J.T. Marsh, S. Greenberg, and W.S. Brown. "Human Auditory Frequency-Following Responses to a Missing Fundamental." *Science* 201 (1975): 639–641.

Vanderwolf, C.H. "Are Neocortical Gamma Waves Related to Consciousness?." *Brain Research* 855 (2000): 217–24.

Wagner, U.; S. Gais, H. Haider, R. Verleger, and J. Born. "Sleep Inspires Insight." *Nature* 427 (2004): 352–5.

Chapter 10: Sleep (Get More!)

Benedict, C. and et al., "Acute sleep deprivation increases serum levels of neuron-specific enolase (NSE) and S100 calcium binding protein B (S-100B) in healthy young men." *SLEEP* (2013).

Aho, Vilma, M. Hanna, Ville Rantanen Ollila, Erkki Kronholm, et al. "Partial Sleep Restriction Activates Immune Response-Related Gene Expression Pathways: Experimental and Epidemiological Studies in Humans." *Public Library of Science* 8 (2013): e77184.

Anch, A.M., C.P. Browman, M.M. Mitler, and J.K. Walsh. *Sleep: A Scientific Perspective*. Englewood Cliffs, N.J.: Prentice Hall, 1988.

Webb, W.B. and M.G. Dube. "Temporal Characteristics of Sleep." *Handbook of Behavioral Neurobiology* (1981): 510–517.

Born, Jan, Kirsten Hansen, Lisa Marshall, Matthias Mölle, and Horst L. Fehm. "Timing the End of Nocturnal Sleep." *Nature* 397 (1999): 29–30.

Gupta, P.D. and K. Pushkala. "Prevalence of Breast Cancer in Pre and Postmenopausal Blind Women." *Advances in Medical and Dental Sciences* 3(2009): 40–45.

Pace-Schott, Edward F. *Sleep and Dreaming: Scientific Advances and Reconsiderations.* Cambridge, Mass.: Cambridge University Press, 2003.

Broussard, Josiane L., David A. Ehrmann, Eve Van Cauter, Esra Tasali, and Matthew J. Brady. "Impaired Insulin Signaling in Human Adipocytes after Experimental Sleep Restriction: A Randomized, Crossover Study." *Annals of Internal Medicine* 157 (2012): 549–5.

Appendix

LeBlanc, Erin S. MD, MPH, Joanne H. Rizzo, MPA, M.S. Pedula, L. Kathryn, et al. "The Endocrine Society's Clinical Guidelines for the Evaluation, Treatment and Prevention of Vitamin D Deficiency." *Journal of Clinical Endocrinology & Metabolism* 96 (2011): 1911–1930.

Index

Index

About the Author

Jeanne Ricks, CHC, has a passion for teaching and sharing information about how we can all optimize our health and improve our sense of well-being. As former director of Holistic Wellness Programs for City College of New York, she developed programs that emphasize self-healing through nutrition, breathing techniques, and meditation; self-empowerment through practical techniques for coping with stress and building health and vitality; and developing inner resources to confront adversity and challenges in one's life. Her outreach not only empowers the average person, but also reaches those battling alcoholism, drug addiction, domestic violence, mental illness, and the isolation often experienced by the elderly. She is an independent holistic health counselor, lecturer, and life coach whose motto is "As we instill new ideas, behavior changes, health improves."

Her websites are: *www.NuDay.org* and *www.VibroAcousticNY.com*